'For many practitioners, working with bilingual children can seem daunting. This book goes a long way towards dispelling such worries by providing detailed practical information and guidance on how to proceed while also giving clear explanations as to why certain approaches should be taken. Examples of assessment pro-formas, questionnaires and charts (for example for working out the amount of interpreter time needed) are provided which should be invaluable. Additionally, it is recognised that many SLTs will work in situations where providing an equitable service is challenging; the book empowers practitioners to fight for necessary resources within the context of current societal issues around diversity, equality, and racism.'

**Carolyn Letts**, *Senior Research Investigator, Newcastle University*

'This timely and important book should be read by all paediatric Speech and Language Therapists/Speech Pathologists in practice and in training. In "Working with Children Experiencing Speech and Language Disorders in a Bilingual Context: A home language approach" Dr Sean Pert provides extensive and highly practical advice for clinical practice covering issue of assessment, diagnosis and intervention in language and speech sound disorders. Importantly this book unpacks aspects of best practice which are rarely documented, such as working with interpreters and the use of AAC for languages other than English when many systems and devices are designed with English only in mind.

Perhaps most important however is the powerful challenge Dr Pert poses our profession to acknowledge the uncomfortable truth that much of our current practice for bilingual families is systematically and institutionally racist. Together with an analysis of the barriers which need to be overcome and a call for anti-racist and culturally inquisitive practice this book provides the profession with a platform and tools to move forward towards equity and social justice for children experiencing Speech and Language Disorders in a Bilingual Context.'

**Cristina McKean**, BSc MSc PhD, *Professor of Child Language Development and Disorders, Newcastle University*

# Access your online resources

*Working with Children Experiencing Speech and Language Disorders in a Bilingual Context* is accompanied by a number of printable online materials, designed to ensure this resource best supports your professional needs

Activate your online resources:

Go to www.routledge.com/cw/speechmark and click on the cover of this book

Click the "Sign in or Request Access" button and follow the instructions in order to access the resources

# Working with Children Experiencing Speech and Language Disorders in a Bilingual Context

The complexity of speech and language disorders can be daunting in a monolingual context. When working with a bilingual child assessment and intervention may appear to be even more complicated. In this book Sean Pert provides the reader with the tools needed to overcome this perception and develop skills in working in a language that they don't share with the client.

By adopting a home language first approach the book discusses how to:

- identify diversity from disorder
- introduce effective approaches in line with the best clinical practice
- work successfully alongside interpreters
- make assessments and plan interventions
- set goals for therapy.

At the heart of the text is the therapist creating essential partnerships with parents and truly valuing the bilingualism, culture, and identity of the child. This leads to better outcomes, not only in speech, language, and communication, but also in self-esteem, mental health, social participation, and educational and employment success.

The book concludes with a handy toolkit of resources including quizzes, case studies and printable extras making it the perfect resource for both experienced and newly qualified practitioners with bilingual and multilingual children in their care.

**Sean Pert** (he/him) worked in the NHS for almost 20 years, in one of the few departments to deliver a speech and language therapy service exclusively in the family's home language or mother tongue. He provided a service to children with the most severe and complex speech and language disorders and shares his specialist knowledge as a trainer both in the UK and internationally. He is currently a Senior Clinical Lecturer at the University of Manchester, and a Consultant Speech and Language Therapist. A three-times joint winner of the Sternberg Award for Clinical Innovation, Sean is the Service Lead for the Voice and Communication Therapy Team, Indigo Gender Service, and Chair of the Board for the Royal College of Speech and Language Therapists. See his full biography at www.research. manchester.ac.uk/portal/sean.pert.html

## The *Working With* Series

The *Working With* series provides speech and language therapists with a range of 'go-to' resources, full of well-sourced, up-to-date information regarding specific disorders. Underpinned by robust theoretical foundations and supported by intervention options and exercises, every book ensures that the reader has access to the latest thinking regarding diagnosis, management and treatment options.

Written in a fully accessible style, each book bridges theory and practice and offers ready-to-use and well-rehearsed practical material, including guidance on interventions, management advice, and therapeutic resources for the client, parent or carer. The series is an invaluable resource for practitioners, whether speech and language therapy students, or more experienced clinicians.

Books in the series include:

*Working with Children's Language*, 2nd edition
Diana Williams
2022 / pb: 9780367467913

*Working with Voice Disorders: Theory and Practice*, 3rd edition
Stephanie Martin
2021 / pb: 9780863889462

*Working with Communication and Swallowing Difficulties in Older Adults*
Rebecca Allwood
2022 / pb: 9780367524784

*Working with Solution Focused Brief Therapy in Healthcare Settings*
Kidge Burns and Sarah Northcott
2022 / pb: 9780367435097

*Working with Children Experiencing Speech and Language Disorders in a Bilingual Context*
Sean Pert
2022 / pb: 9780367646301

*Working with Global Aphasia*
Sharon Adjei-Nicol
2023 / pb: 9781032019437

*Working with Trans Voice*
Matthew Mills and Sean Pert
2023 / pb: 9781032012605

# Working with Children Experiencing Speech and Language Disorders in a Bilingual Context

## A Home Language Approach

**Sean Pert**

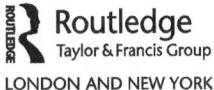
Routledge
Taylor & Francis Group

LONDON AND NEW YORK

Cover image: Illustration by Reyyan Hammad, BA (2022)

First published 2023
by Routledge
4 Park Square, Milton Park, Abingdon, Oxon OX14 4RN

and by Routledge
605 Third Avenue, New York, NY 10158

*Routledge is an imprint of the Taylor & Francis Group, an informa business*

*British Library Cataloguing-in-Publication Data*
A catalogue record for this book is available from the British Library

*Library of Congress Cataloging-in-Publication Data*
Names: Pert, Sean, author.
Title: Working with children experiencing speech and language disorders in a bilingual context : a home language approach / Sean Pert.
Description: First edition. | Abingdon, Oxon ; New York, NY : Routledge, 2023. | Series: Working with ; 5 | Includes bibliographical references and index.
Identifiers: LCCN 2022023957 (print) | LCCN 2022023958 (ebook) | ISBN 9780367646356 (hbk) | ISBN 9780367646301 (pbk) | ISBN 9781003125563 (ebk)
Subjects: LCSH: Speech disorders in children. | Language disorders in children. | Bilingualism in children.
Classification: LCC RJ496.S7 P425 2023 (print) | LCC RJ496.S7 (ebook) | DDC 618.92/855—dc23/eng/20220809
LC record available at https://lccn.loc.gov/2022023957
LC ebook record available at https://lccn.loc.gov/2022023958

ISBN: 978-0-367-64635-6 (hbk)
ISBN: 978-0-367-64630-1 (pbk)
ISBN: 978-1-003-12556-3 (ebk)

DOI: 10.4324/9781003125563

Typeset in Interstate
by Apex CoVantage, LLC

Access the companion website: www.routledge.com/cw/speechmark

For my mother, Bettina Sandra Richards,

who knew coal mining wasn't for me.

# Contents

# Contributors

**Suzanne Martin,** Speech and Language Therapist and Senior AAC Consultant at ACE Centre, UK.

**Lizzie Sadiku,** Speech and Language Therapist and AAC Consultant at Ace Centre, UK.

**Katherine Small,** Speech and Language Therapist and AAC Consultant at Ace Centre, UK.

**Ace Centre** is a registered charity (No. 1089313) providing Assistive Technology and Augmentative and Alternative Communication services for people with complex needs. https://acecentre.org.uk

**Carol Stow** is a retired Consultant Speech and Language Therapist in Bilingualism, and pioneer of a mother tongue children's speech and language therapy service in Rochdale, Greater Manchester, UK.

# Tables

# Figures

# Preface

This book is a result of my professional encounters with bilingual families with speech, language, and communication disorders. This work can be daunting, as the speech and language therapist is faced with working with different families speaking tens or even hundreds of languages within one geographical area. It would be easy to give up and say, "What choice do I have but to use only the mainstream language, English?" That would not only be a shame for the children and young people, who, being assessed and treated exclusively in English (or mainstream language) will almost inevitably lose their home language through language attrition, but also a missed opportunity for the clinician themselves.

As a clinician I have learnt so much about the value of culture, and how language is the way that culture is transmitted to children, allowing them to share in the cultural wealth of their community. Isolation from your home language is to be isolated from your family, religion, and heritage, isolation from your own identity. To maintain your home language and confidently gain an additional language or develop the two (or more) languages together is to become a fully rounded individual with the tools to enjoy an engaging life across your cultures.

As a white, working-class monolingual child and young person, I did not encounter bilingualism until as a young adult I moved from a small mining town to large cities in the UK. Here I encountered difficult cultures and languages for the first time. I was possibly the least likely person to develop a special interest in bilingualism and cultures. I have been fortunate to work professionally with many skilled bilingual professionals, and to slowly develop my own bilingual skills. I am now able to speak some basic Mirpuri (a Pakistani-heritage language), much to the amusement of my young service users, who think that a white man speaking their language is so unusual that it is unvaryingly hilarious! While appearing on a Community Radio show, some callers refused to believe that a white English speaker could use the Mirpuri language so well. Although flattered that my pronunciation was so accurate, this demonstrates the gulf between two communities living in the same town. It also demonstrates that professionals are often white and monolingual, that bilingual people don't expect monolingual people to make the effort to learn their language and culture, and that bilingual communities often face barriers entering healthcare professions such as speech and language therapy.

I hope that this book encourages people of colour and bilingual speakers to consider speech and language therapy as a career, and that white monolingual clinicians use their professional privilege to ensure that home language services are made available, and that Black, Asian, and people of different ethnicities are supported and encouraged in their careers.

# Acknowledgements

This book is dedicated to the Bilingual Speech and Language Therapy Team of which I was fortunate enough to be a member. The team was built up by Dr Carol Stow, FRCSLT, Consultant Speech and Language Therapist (Retired). Carol had insight into the institutional racism prevalent in the UK in the 1990s and 2000s and provided a high-quality service for families who spoke languages other than English. Carol built up a team of three specialist speech and language therapists and six bilingual speech and language therapy assistants or bilingual co-workers. The team worked alongside interpreters to ensure that all families received assessment and therapy in their home language(s). This award-winning team are a model for services where bilingual families receive a truly equitable and welcoming provision.

I would like to thank the following people for all their help and support in the development of this book:

- **Dr Carol Stow**, FRCSLT, Consultant Speech and Language Therapist (Retired)
- **Zahida Warriach**, Senior Bilingual Speech and Language Therapy Assistant
- **Carly Hartshorn**, Clinical Lead Speech and Language Therapist
- **Katherine Small, Lizzie Sadiku and Suzanne Martin,** AAC Consultants, Ace Centre, UK
- All the children, young people and families who have accessed the service over the years for being so open and generous in sharing their experiences.

I would also like to thank the late **Sandra J. Robertson** for encouraging me to undertake a career in speech and language therapy. As well as Programme Director for the BSc (Hons) Speech and Language Pathology degree programme, Sandra was the Chair of the Royal College of Speech and Language Therapists when I was just commencing my degree. Sandra was also the author of the pioneering *Working with Dysarthrics: A Practical Guide to Therapy for Dysarthria* (1986) and *The Robertson Dysarthria Profile* (1982). I am delighted to honour her memory by treading the same path.

## References

Robertson, S. J., & Thomson, F. (1986). *Working with dysarthrics: A practical guide to therapy for dysarthria*. Speechmark.

Robertson, S. J. (1982). *Dysarthria profile*. Winslow Press.

# Acronyms and abbreviations

| | |
|---|---|
| **AAC** | Augmentative and Alternative Communication |
| **ASHA** | American Speech-Language-Hearing Association |
| **Cis** | The person's presenting gender is the same as the sex that they were assigned at birth |
| **COVID-19** | Coronavirus disease caused by severe acute respiratory syndrome coronavirus 2 (SARS-CoV-2) |
| **CPD** | Continuing Professional Development |
| **CV** | Consonant + Vowel, such as [ki] |
| **VC** | Vowel + Consonant, such as [ik] |
| **CVC** | Consonant + Vowel + Consonant, such as [tik] |
| **DLD** | Developmental Language Disorder |
| **LGBTQ+** | Lesbian, Gay, Bisexual, Trans(gender), Queer, and other self-defined labels (+) referring to an individual's sexuality, gender, and identity |
| **LOTE** | Language(s) Other Than English |
| **PBUH** | A benediction used by Muslim people meaning "Peace be upon him" when referring to the Prophet, as a sign of respect |
| **RCSLT** | Royal College of Speech and Language Therapists |
| **SLT** | Speech and Language Therapist |
| **SSD** | Speech Sound Disorder |
| **SES** | Socioeconomic status |
| **TPOC** | Trans people of colour |
| **Trans** | an umbrella term referring to any person who does not identify with the sex assigned at birth. This includes trans(gender), gender diverse and non-binary people |

# 1

# INTRODUCTION

DOI: 10.4324/9781003125563-1

## Introduction

This book is aimed at SLTs (UK, New Zealand, South Africa), also known as speech and language pathologists (SLPs) (US, Australia) and Logopèdes/Logopèdistes/Orthophonistes (European countries), specialist teachers, students, and other professions working with children acquiring two or more languages and who are also experiencing speech, language, and communication disorders.

Children who are exposed to two or more languages, or who are raised in a home where a language that is different to the mainstream language is used are just as likely as monolingual children to experience speech and language disorders (Stow & Dodd, 2005; Crutchley et al., 1997).

The complexity of speech and language disorders can be daunting in a monolingual context and may *appear* to be an even bigger challenge in a bilingual context. I use the term "appear," because bilingual children are just as likely to experience speech and language disorders as their monolingual peers, and the complexity is for us as professionals. The vast majority of SLTs in the UK are white monolingual English speakers (Moore et al., 2020) and so will not share a language or cultural perspective with their client. Even for those SLTs who are bilingual and can work with two or three speech communities, they cannot hope to speak the tens or hundreds of diverse languages commonly encountered on a caseload. Working in a language we do not share with our client is therefore a skill all professionals working with bilingual families will need.

It is important to note that this is *not* a guide on raising typically developing children in a bilingual environment, or children who have acquired a home language with no difficulties and are in the early stages of acquiring an additional language. The vast majority of bilingual children go on to acquire their additional language (and indeed other additional languages) with no extra help from professionals. Bilingualism is the normal human condition, and there is no evidence that bilingualism causes or contributes to any speech, language, or communication disorder. The false belief that bilingualism itself causes a child any difficulties in acquiring speech and language skills and should be considered a disorder is derived from an exclusively monolingual perspective, and a racist assumption that bilingualism is unusual, outside the monolingual "norm" or "other" in some way. There is no evidence to support this view and SLTs and other professionals should therefore *never* recommend giving up speaking the home language(s) to support additional language acquisition.

The profession has a responsibility to address the inherent racism and "othering" of speakers of home languages, or mother tongue languages. Most speech and language therapy programmes teach exclusively from the monolingual (mainly English) perspective. There is rarely teaching on, for example, Speech Sound Disorders, from a bilingual or multilingual perspective, or using examples from languages other than English. This has led to the false view that English is the "default" language. This view is institutionally racist and continues to fail both bilingual individuals and communities. Our profession has a history of both over-referral and under-referral of bilingual children to specialist provisions (Crutchley, 2000). Children from other cultures, especially Black children, have been incorrectly diagnosed with language disorders or learning difficulties due to biased assessment materials that dismiss linguistic diversity as disorder (BBC, 2021).

The NHS has consistently failed in its duty to address racism, with managers and team leads often incorrectly and illegally minimising the need for interpreters on the basis of cost. In 2022 a report stated that systemic failures including inequitable treatment from staff had led to negative outcomes for service users. Factors identified highlighted a "lack of appropriate interpreting services for people who do not speak English confidently and delays in, or avoidance of, seeking help for health problems due to fear of racist treatment from NHS healthcare professionals." (Kapadia et al., 2022, p. 10).

This book is aimed primarily at the white monolingual SLT. Those who are bilingual, or from non-white cultures will already be familiar with the extreme bias against other languages and cultures. If the text in this book speaks to the monolingual (usually white) SLT, I make no apology. To be an ally and address these biases and prejudices, those with the power to do so must carry out the work to become aware of these biases and prejudices. More importantly, becoming educated about the barriers bilingual families face helps us to advocate for bilingual families and facilitate better outcomes where home language(s) and cultures are prioritised.

This is not just political correctness. The impact of losing home language is real and harmful. Loss of home language, or mother tongue is often a cause of regret, even mourning.

> And now my mother is dead, and I do not speak the language she spoke, and I feel I have lost not just my mother, but half my heritage, too. You can never understand a country if you don't speak the language.
>
> (Patterson, 2019)

Children can be severed from their families, extended communities and even their own parents.

> I think the saddest part is even not going to grandparents. Some young people can't converse with their own parents, because they don't know the language.
>
> *Zahida Warriach, Multilingual speaker, parent of bilingual children*
> *and bilingual professional.*

In the UK the Royal College of Speech and Language Therapists is attempting to address the lack of diversity in the profession and to decolonise the curriculum in pre-qualification programmes in universities. This essential work seeks to align the profession so that it is more representative of the population we serve.

## The impact of COVID-19

The evidence about the impact of the COVID-19 pandemic is still emerging. However, what is clear is that the pandemic has exacerbated inequalities and affected those who are poor or discriminated against even more than pre-pandemic. Even prior to the pandemic, ethnic minority populations were more likely to live in poverty. In the UK, "employment rates among white British individuals are 73 per cent for women and 80 per cent for men, but among Pakistanis and Bangladeshis they are 39 per cent and 75 per cent respectively" (Blundell et al., 2020, p. 294).

Children received less speech and language therapy during lockdown, with a resulting negative impact on education, social life and mental health (Clegg et al., 2021). Many children face longer waiting times as services address backlogs, with later diagnosis leading to poorer outcomes for those with Developmental Language Disorder and other conditions (Royal College of Speech and Language Therapists, 2022).

A small but significant number of children will experience COVID-19 syndrome or "Long COVID" (Ashkenazi-Hoffnung et al., 2021) and may require speech and language therapy as part of their rehabilitation.

One of the impacts of the COVID-19 was the dramatic increase in telehealth as a means of delivering assessment, advice, and intervention. Familiarity with this method of service delivery increased in both service users and practitioners, since this was the only possible method available when lockdowns mandated the families stay at home (Royal College of Speech and Language Therapists, 2022). For some families, the involvement of interpreters over telehealth video calls may have made access to home language support more convenient. However, many families will have barriers to accessing telehealth due to the costs of internet connection and associated hardware.

## Speech and language disorders

Difficulties acquiring speech and language is the most common childhood disability. These domains are therefore the focus of this book. It is common for more than one difficulty to be present (co-morbidity), and a full assessment of the child's abilities should be completed prior to setting therapy aims and commencing intervention.

This book does not have sufficient space to explore in depth many important communities, themes, and topics, including dysphagia, Deaf and hearing-impaired people, sign language, and bilingualism where an individual has learning difficulties, is autistic/has autism, and many other diverse individuals. Bilingual people and families are just as likely to have the same range of needs, conditions, and differences as monolingual people. For this I apologise. However, the reader can be assured that the same principle of home language first applies.

SLTs should work holistically. Only by addressing all the languages the child or young person hears and/or speaks is a holistic approach possible. Many people have tried to argue that assessments and interventions can be delivered in only one language (and this language is usually the language of education, and most frequently English in the UK). This position ignores the harmful message that this conveys to families; that their home language(s) are not important or valuable. Even if this approach were possible (which I argue against in this book), the implementation of a monolingual language of education approach fails to value bilingualism and the family's culture and identity. This is why a *home language first approach* is recommended. Language is inextricably entwined with culture and without home language children and young people are cut off from their relatives and wider community and all the emotional and cultural riches they provide.

## The practicality of a home language first approach

SLTs may feel that they work with such a diverse range of languages and cultures that a home language first approach is not practical. I am confidently able to refute this claim. I spend many years working in a service in the North West of England where all assessment and therapy was in home language. The ground-breaking service was established by Dr Carol Stow, FRCSLT, Consultant Speech and Language Therapist (Retired). She not only established a service where all assessments and therapy packages were delivered in home language(s) but established that this approach provided excellent outcomes. Children and young people attending the service not only improved their speech and language but went on to become successful additional language speakers while retaining and developing their home language skills. Waiting lists were comparable with other services. This book owes a great deal to her vision of a fair and equitable service for bilingual children and their families.

Many SLTs imagine that they do not have the skills to work in a language they do not share with a client. SLTs are uniquely placed to assess children and young people. They are trained in phonetic transcription, have training on phonology and linguistics and have insight into pragmatics and other important areas of communication. Working alongside an interpreter, SLTs can discover how to assist bilingual children presenting with speech, language, and communication needs. Crucially, this will involve seeking information on the language(s) in the home, as well as time to assess and plan the child or young person's needs with the interpreter. This will take at least double the time compared to working with a child or young person who shares your language. The outcomes of home language working involve the retention of home language and culture. This outcome supports the development of identity and good mental health. This outcome is therefore always superior to an additional language (typically monolingual English) approach.

This book considers a home language(s) first approach, in contrast to a bilingual approach to intervention. This is a clinical approach designed to support home language(s) which are often viewed negatively and highly likely to be lost through language attrition.

## Mirpuri, a Pakistani-heritage language

Many of the examples cited are from Pakistani-heritage families, the largest ethnic minority group in Manchester, UK (Khan, 2011). Readers should note that most speakers from this community speak **Mirpuri** (also known as Pahari, Kashmiri, Mirpuri Pahari, Mirpuri Punjabi or Mirpuri Pothowari) originating "from the Mirpur District of Pakistan-administered Jammu and Kashmir" (Hussain, 2015, p. 484). This language is often conflated with Punjabi but is linguistically distinct. Some members of the Pakistani-heritage community in the UK also speak Punjabi and/or Urdu, although it should be noted that the variant of Punjabi is distinct from Indian Panjabi (Jackson, 1987). Mirpuri is often overlooked in the UK and incorrectly considered to be a mutually intelligible dialect of Punjabi or Urdu.

## Acknowledging and valuing linguistic diversity in the profession

In this book I will mainly discuss the perspective of the monolingual SLT who speaks English as their first language and has little or no knowledge of other languages. It is important to acknowledge that although this is the situation for most of the profession, there will of course be SLTs and SLT assistants who speak languages other than English (LOTE). Such individuals are highly valuable members of the team. Bilingual professionals are able to bring insights into different cultures, attitudes to child-rearing, attitudes to disability, religious beliefs, and the experience of using a language other than English.

There are also speech communities both in the UK, the US, and Europe where languages other than English are the main language. In other communities there will be different attitudes and frequency of use of particular languages. It is not possible within the confines of this book to write a text that covers every possible eventuality. It is therefore important to bear in mind that the main thrust of this text is to support the family to be confident in using their home language. This approach means that the home language will not suffer attrition causing later difficulties with cultural identity and loss of cultural diversity within both the family and the wider community.

Important examples in the UK include Welsh speaking communities, where Welsh may be the community language as well as the language of education, Gaelic language speakers in Scotland, as well as communities that speak languages from many parts of the globe. Immigration has led to a multicultural society where many languages and cultures may be encountered in towns and cities. This cultural richness is in constant flux. Some families may adopt the mainstream language and become monolingual. Other families may maintain their home language to varying degrees. Contact between community languages and the mainstream language is likely to result in codeswitched varieties of languages.

In many communities in the US Spanish predominates as a community language and there are many texts and research papers exploring the specific challenges of home language speakers within these communities.

Bilingual staff may or may not wish to work with bilingualism as their primary specialist interest. In my career I have encountered bilingual SLTs who have been expected to work with bilingual communities simply because they are themselves bilingual. Such bilingual speech language therapists may wish to work within other specialist areas and should not be expected or pressured to work exclusively in the bilingual field.

Additionally, just because a person can work with two or more languages does not mean that they have insight into other speech communities. As a result, SLTs, including bilingual SLTs, will need the skill of working alongside a professional interpreter to meet the needs of the whole community.

SLTs who speak a language other than English to a native level should be encouraged to work with their speech community if they wish to do so. Each speech language therapist is responsible for evaluating their own clinical and linguistic skill level in relation to a particular family and client. If a professional feels that they are competent to work in a language other than English, then they will not need to work alongside a professional interpreter for that particular language.

Examples provided in this book focus on the English monolingual SLT or a bilingual SLT working in a language they do not share with the client and family.

## Gaining confidence in working in Languages Other Than English (LOTE)

A monolingual English-speaking SLT has immediate access to examples of grammatical utterances in that language and can identify words that start/contain/end with a particular phone. As an experienced SLT, I can often hear children in the waiting room. Listening to their speech during play I immediately begin to identify speech errors and errors and omissions in their spoken utterances. It is not until we are faced with a family who do not use English that we start to reflect on how much automatic analysis we undertake.

So, how can we develop confidence when working with families who speak languages other than English (LOTE)? SLTs are encouraged to take a lifelong learning approach to their career. Developing new skills takes time and during this development process SLTs should liaise with more experienced colleagues to discuss cases in clinical supervision. In addition, SLTs have access to evidence based clinical guidelines from both the Royal College of Speech and Language Therapists (RCSLT) and the American Speech and Hearing Association (ASHA).

Setting learning goals, shadowing SLTs who work in languages other than English, shadowing sessions led by a therapist working alongside a professional interpreter, reading about the development of a particular language, and finding out about other cultures are key to developing confidence in this field. In addition to double the time taken when working in a language you do not share with the client, it is also important to take time to reflect and identify when practice has gone well and when things may need adjusting for future practice. Reflection has been shown to improve clinical practice and should be a valued part of any SLT's development.

SLTs wishing to develop their skills should plan to present case studies to their peers at clinical excellence network meetings, conferences, and panels. It is often mentioned that professionals working with families from a different culture to their own should strive to develop cultural competence. I do not think that it is possible to be completely culturally *competent* in a culture that one does not live day by day. The insights from lived experience are impossible to replicate by continual professional development alone. However, we can strive to be culturally *inquisitive*. This means being open to the idea that people with a culture we do not share have different ways of carrying out their lives. This will include attitudes, beliefs, and ways of being. The professional should take the approach that people from cultures different to our own may do things in a different but equally valid manner.

## Racism in the profession and internalised racism

The recent heightened awareness of racist attitudes to cultures other than western culture has highlighted that racism and negative attitudes to people from other cultures is commonly encountered. Colonialism has resulted in centuries of denigration of peoples across the globe and it will take a great deal of effort and will to reverse ingrained attitudes towards non-western cultures. Casual racism, failing to value people's language and culture, micro aggressions and other forms of racism can have a major negative impact on families. Families may feel unable to access services, or fear that revealing their use of home language will result in censure from monolingual professionals. This is especially true when children have a diagnosis such as Developmental Language Disorder (DLD) or other long-term or severe condition.

Individuals, and indeed whole services may not view themselves as racist, but the experience of families may be quite different. Structural and procedural barriers can exist that inadvertently exclude families who speak languages other than English. Examples include advertising the service using pictures featuring only white monolingual families, only providing information about the service in (written) English and no other languages, and only providing assessment and intervention in English (or the language of education such as Welsh). These and many other barriers may be identified and eliminated by the involvement of bilingual families in the design and review of speech language therapy services.

Co-production is essential to ensuring that services are accessible by all members of the community.

It is not uncommon to encounter families where parent(s)/carer(s) have absorbed racist attitudes towards their language and culture so that they have highly negative perspectives about their own language usage. This internalised racism is an inevitable consequence of living in a society which is inherently racist. SLTs must actively challenge these negative attitudes and support families to see that using their own language and valuing their home culture will not lead to poor outcomes for their child. Many families will fear that speaking their own language and not the language of education will slow their child's ability to engage with the education system. Since education is a key route that people from all backgrounds can improve their access to employment, this concern is understandable. SLTs have an important role in educating parents and carers that speaking the home language well not impair a child's ability to learn English nor will it affect their educational outcome.

Mandatory training on both explicit and implicit racism and bias are highly recommended. Annual updates, and reviews of the service by families from a co-production panel and/or advisory panel are also effective ways of ensuring the service remains open and welcoming to all.

## Diversity and families: LGBTQ+

Diversity is not limited to ethnicity and cultural differences. Intersectionality is an important consideration when working with diverse families. Class, race, gender, sexuality, and many other aspects of our individual make-up need to be considered when establishing good working relationships and trust with families (see Choudrey, 2022).

Many services, especially those aimed at children and young people are constructed to assume that parents will be heterosexual and cisgender. This can act as a barrier to accessing services. Same-sex families, trans and non-binary parents and young people, and indeed SLTs and other professionals from LGBTQ+ communities need representation, staff, and services to ensure that they are included. Twenty-three per cent of LGBTQ+ people have witnessed homo/bi/trans/phobic remarks by professionals when accessing healthcare (Bachmann & Gooch, 2018).

Questions on interview proformas/templates (case history, reports, advice leaflets) should not include stereotyped roles and terminology that makes assumptions. Terms such as

"Parent/carer 01" and "Parent/carer 02" should be used in the first instance, rather than "Mother" and "Father." This not only makes services welcoming and accessible for LGBTQ+ families, but also ensures single-parent families, foster care, and other family structures are welcomed within your service.

Some practitioners may argue that this is an erasure of important terms such as "Mother" and "Father." Not so! This is not about enforcing generic terms on anyone. Rather, it is having the courtesy to specifically ask names that are used within the family. Many same-sex families use the term "Mother" or "Father."

Cis-heterosexual families may also have family circumstances where an open questioning approach is more sensitive than making assumptions. Families where parents have separated but are both still involved in the care of the child(ren) need an opportunity to explain how their pattern of care is implemented. The SLT might ask:

"Who will attend appointments with the child?" and get the reply

"It might be his mum, dad, or older step-brother . . . their names and contact details are . . ."

This is much more helpful than challenging the child's stepbrother when he attends clinic with the child and staff do not recognise him!

Many trans and non-binary young people and adults relate contact with services when they were children that were negative experiences. This may make these individuals far less likely to access vital services in the future. Consideration of materials, especially around pronouns and depictions of gender roles should be made. Are your therapy materials highly binary?

Finally, representation is important. Posters and leaflets for services should be inclusive whilst avoiding tokenism. Auditing services, and a co-production approach to the development of assessment and therapy materials with service users from the LGBTQ+ community will help you to identify where changes need to be made.

## Professional power and privilege

SLTs are professions with a great deal of power and privilege. We can diagnose, recommend, and deliver treatment, refer on to other professionals, and decide levels of support. Qualified SLTs are educated to degree level or above, meaning that they have received many years of education. Such professionals take being able to read for granted, for example. Many of our service users will have been held back or prevented from reaching their potential by discrimination and exclusion.

As professionals we can choose to use our power and privilege to recognise the overt and subconscious barriers our services have, and work to address these. We can empower students and our colleagues to educate themselves about bilingualism and build a more inclusive set of care pathways and services.

Alternatively, we can choose to minimise the need to preserve and develop bilingualism. You may find yourself thinking the following things, or hear colleagues saying something similar:

- "It is easier and more convenient to work in my language." (most frequently English)
- "I dislike working via an interpreter. They might be late, and it takes much longer than working just in English!"
- "Interpreters cost too much. We don't provide a 'Gold Standard'"
- "We should treat everyone the same way. That means speaking English (or Welsh) and not taking more time to involve an interpreter."
- "Families living in this country should speak English/Welsh anyway. I'm helping the child to integrate."
- "The child/young person has almost lost their home language, so why bother?"
- "The child/young person speaks in English at school, so does it matter if they don't use their home language?"

All these statements and questions lead to a single outcome: The child or young person loses their home language (language attrition) and is isolated from their family, extended family, and community.

If you are an English speaker, or Welsh speaker, or speaker of a privileged language with a written form and rich culture, you would not tolerate this attitude to your own language. You would not live in another country and accept that you should stop speaking English at home and allow your child to lose their English ability. Why do we expect speakers of other languages to accept this racist nonsense?

## My personal perspective

I am now a white middle class man living in northern England, UK. I work as a Senior Lecturer at the University of Manchester. Manchester is one of the most diverse cities in the UK, with an estimated 300+ languages spoken.

I grew up in a small coal mining town in the East Midlands in a working-class mining village and nearby town. As such, I had little to no contact with people of colour when growing up, and certainly didn't encounter bilingual people. I never heard anyone speak another language. As part of a working-class family, I did not have access to books unless they were in my local library. The internet was decades from being invented. My experience of Modern Foreign Languages was an hour or two of German lessons from the age of 11 to the age of 16. Our language laboratory had no working audio facilities, and the textbooks were many years old.

As a student, I moved firstly to Birmingham and then to Manchester, England. These hugely diverse cities meant that I encountered children, young people, and adults from many different cultural and linguistic backgrounds.

On qualifying, I was fortunate to find employment as a SLT in a small post-industrial town in the North West of England. This town had a sizable bilingual community, consisting of Pakistani- and Bangladeshi-heritage people who were invited to work in the town's cotton mills from the 1950s onwards, as well as people from all over the world, as the town was also a centre for families with both asylum seeker and refugee status. More recent economic migration saw families from Eastern European counties such as Poland move to the town.

The opportunity to consider developing better, culturally appropriate assessment tools and therapy equipment came about as I worked in a thriving bilingual team led by Dr Carol Stow. We developed culturally sensitive photo cards featuring food, drinks, everyday objects, and local people. We then moved onto the development of an informal speech sound assessment in Pakistani-heritage languages.

This led to a meeting with Dr Alison Holm, a Speech Pathologist who was conducting research into Speech Sound Disorder in languages other than English. We were convinced by Professor Barbara Dodd who was supervising Alison's PhD to undertake PhD studies, Carol on speech sound assessment and me on language assessment. This ultimately led to the development of the *Bilingual Speech Sound Screen for Pakistani heritage languages* (BiSSS) (Stow & Pert, 2020) and the *Bilingual Assessment of Simple Sentences* (BASS) (Pert & Stow, 2019). Carol and I attended many conferences both within the UK and internationally as part of our studies.

Carol wrote some of the first evidence-based professional guidelines on bilingualism for the Royal College of Speech and Language Therapists (RCSLT) for the various iterations of

*Communicating Quality.* I had the honour of updating these recently for the RCSLT website. It was gratifying to see that the core messages of home language assessment and therapy being central to effective care was still at the heart of these guidelines.

I have been involved in the Language Intervention in the Early Years (LIVELY) randomised control trial. This project, led by Professor Cristina McKean, will "evaluate the effectiveness of language interventions for pre-school children in nursery contexts with significant language difficulties" (McKean et al., 2020). One of the interventions being investigated in the Building Early Sentences Therapy (BEST) (McKean et al., 2010) To demonstrate that the approach is suitable for languages other than English, I have been involved in the adaptation of the BEST materials and other assessments into Polish, Mirpuri, a Pakistani-heritage language, and Sylheti, a Bangladeshi-heritage language.

My approach, along with colleagues that have been successful in developing culturally appropriate and linguistically sensitive assessment and therapy materials involves:

- Prioritising home language
- Co-production with people from the community who speak the language
- Consulting several adult informants
- Working with professional interpreters
- Combining linguistic knowledge with practical usage, for example accepting borrowings and codeswitching where these have become the dominant form of a word or phrase
- Using pictures, toys and objects that will be recognised by children from the community
- Adapting, *not carrying out a direct translation*, allowing for differences where activities, actions or objects would not be recognised or used by that community or in that particular language.

In my experience, and those who have been successful in working with bilingual families, insisting on best practice is essential to meet the same quality outcomes as when working with monolingual English-speaking families. Compromise on working with professional interpreters for reasons of cost for example, will almost certainly undermine your service and ability to achieve basic differential diagnosis and delivery of home language care.

The most common questions asked by SLTs when I deliver training are:

- Which language should be used to assess and deliver intervention?
- How do we differentiate typical language learning in a bilingual context from speech and Language Difficulties or disorders?

- What is the best way to work with interpreters?

- How can we involve parent(s) and carers who speak no, or little of the mainstream language?

I hope that this book will answer these questions. However, to deliver best practice in a language you do not share with the family, you will need to accept that building trust, experimentation and adaptation of your practice will be required. There are few available published tools, and those that do exist are not available for all language communities. You will need to be inventive, making equipment and collaborating closely with the family. This partnership, co-production and innovation are what makes this work invigorating and exciting. I very much hope that you too will enjoy the challenge of working with children with speech and language disorders in a bilingual context.

## References

Ashkenazi-Hoffnung, L., Shmueli, E., Ehrlich, S., Ziv, A., Bar-On, O., Birk, E., . . . Prais, D. (2021). Long COVID in children: Observations from a designated pediatric clinic. *The Pediatric Infectious Disease Journal, 40*, e509–e511. https://doi.org/10.1097/inf.0000000000003285.

Bachmann, C. L., & Gooch, B. (2018). *LGBT in Britain: Health report*. Stonewall. www.stonewall.org.uk/system/files/lgbt_in_britain_health.pdf

BBC. (2021, May 20). *Subnormal: A British Scandal*. BBC iPlayer. Shannon, L. www.bbc.co.uk/programmes/m000w81h

Blundell, R., Costa Dias, M., Joyce, R., & Xu, X. (2020). COVID-19 and inequalities. *Fiscal Studies, 41*, 291–319. https://doi.org/10.1111/1475-5890.12232

Choudrey, S. (2022). *Supporting trans people of colour*. Jessica Kingsley.

Clegg, J., O'Flynn, P., & Just, P. (2021). *Speech and language therapy during and beyond COVID-19: Building back better with people who have communication and swallowing needs*. Royal College of Speech and Language Therapists. Retrieved February 18, 2021, from www.rcslt.org/wp-content/uploads/2021/03/Building-back-better-March2021.pdf

Crutchley, A. (2000). Bilingual children in language units: Does having 'well informed' parents make a difference? *International Journal of Communication Disorders, 35*, 65–81. https://doi.org/10.1080/136828200247250

Crutchley, A., Conti-Ramsden, G., & Botting, N. (1997). Bilingual children with specific language impairment and standardized assessments: Preliminary findings from a study of children in language units. *International Journal of Bilingualism, 1*, 117–134. https://doi.org/10.1177/136700699700100202

Hussain, S. (2015). Missing from the 'minority mainstream': Pahari-speaking diaspora in Britain. *Journal of Multilingual and Multicultural Development, 36*, 483–497. https://doi.org/10.1080/01434632.2014.953539.

Jackson, H. (1987). The value of error analysis and its implications for teaching and therapy – with special reference to Panjabi learners. In S. Abudarham (Ed.), *Bilingualism and the bilingual*. NFER-NELSON.

Kapadia, D., Zhang, J., Salway, S., Nazroo, J., Booth, A., Villarroel-Williams, N., . . . Esmail, A. (2022). *Ethnic inequalities in healthcare: A rapid evidence review*. NHS Race & Health Observatory. Retrieved February 18, 2022, from www.nhsrho.org/publications/ethnic-inequalities-in-healthcare-a-rapid-evidence-review.

Khan, S. (2011). *Language use and attitudes of the British-born Pakistani community in Manchester*. Bachelor of Arts Dissertation, The University of Manchester. http://www.mlm.humanities.manchester.ac.uk/wp-content/uploads/2015/12/Language-use-and-attitudes-of-the-British-born-Pakistani-community-in-Manchester.pdf

McKean, C., Jack, C., Ashton, E., Preston, E., Benson, K., Rose, N., . . . Trebacz, A. (2020). *Language Intervention in the Early Years (LIVELY)*. Newcastle University. https://www.research.ncl.ac.uk/lively.

McKean, C., Pert, S., & Stow, C. (2010). *Building Early Sentences Therapy (BEST)*. Newcastle University. www.buildingearlysentencestherapy.co.uk

Moore, I., Bitchell, L., & Lord, R. (2020). *The health & care professions council equality, diversity and inclusion data 2020 report*. Health & Care Professions Council. www.hcpc-uk.org/resources/reports/2020/edi-data-2020-report.

Patterson, C. (2019, May 27). I regret not learning my mum's first language. Britain needs those ties. *The Guardian*, Monday. www.theguardian.com/commentisfree/2019/may/27/not-learning-mum-first-language-britain-ties

Pert, S. & Stow, C. (2019). *Bilingual Assessment of Simple Sentences (BASS): An expressive language screening assessment of early sentence production for children with a Pakistani heritage background speaking Mirpuri, Punjabi or Urdu as a home language in the UK*. Royal College of Speech and Language Therapists. www.rcslt.org/members/clinical-guidance/bilingualism/bilingualism-learning/bilingualism-bass

Royal College of Speech and Language Therapists. (2022). *The sustained impact of COVID-19 on speech and language therapy services in the UK*. Royal College of Speech and Language Therapists. Retrieved February 19, 2022, from www.rcslt.org/news/long-covid-and-sustained-impact-reports

Stow, C., & Dodd, B. (2005). A survey of bilingual children referred for investigation of communication disorders: A comparison with monolingual children referred in one area in England. *Journal of Multilingual Communication Disorders, 3*, 1-23. https://doi.org/10.1080/14769670400009959

Stow, C., & Pert, S. (2020). *Bilingual Speech Sound Screen (BiSSS): Revised and expanded edition*. The University of Manchester. https://www.estore.manchester.ac.uk/product-catalogue/faculty-of-biology-medicine-and-health/school-of-health-sciences/bilingual-speech-sound-screen-bisss/bilingual-speech-sound-screen-bisss

# 2

# DEFINITIONS AND TERMINOLOGY

DOI: 10.4324/9781003125563-2

## Bilingualism, Language Disorder and Speech Sound Disorder

This is *not* a book about typical bilingual language acquisition. There are many excellent books and resources available for parents, carers and professionals on supporting typically developing bilingual children (Baker, 2000a, 2000b; Cunningham-Andersson & Andersson, 2004; Myers-Scotton, 2005; Romaine, 1995). It is striking that the consensus view is that home languages/mother tongue in no way impedes children and young people's development of additional/mainstream languages, nor interferes with their ability to access education. It is the ill-informed views of monolingual professionals which need re-balancing through awareness of the evidence.

This book does not attempt to cover all the speech, language, and communication disorders that might be encountered. Bilingual children and young people may experience *any* of the disorders that monolingual people might experience, and the reader is directed to the other books available in this series.

However, it is important to have some basic definitions and concepts around the acquisition of two or more languages. This chapter briefly explores some of the key terms and why they are important when considering if a child or young person presents with a Developmental Language Disorder, Speech Sound Disorder, or is simply a typically developing bilingual child. This is because typical bilingual language acquisition has often been confused with disorder, leading to under- and over-referral and incorrect diagnosis. The most common cause of misdiagnosis is the failure to view the bilingual child holistically. That is, the SLT must have an overview of the child's abilities in both/all languages that they hear or speak. Most SLTs are white monolingual women (Moore et al., 2020), and so an additional language only approach has been the default (most frequently an English only or Welsh-only approach in the UK) due to a complex range of factors including poor access to interpreters, lack of training and under confidence when working in a language the therapist does not share with the family.

Clinical guidelines by both the Royal College of Speech and Language Therapists (Royal College of Speech and Language Therapists, 2019) and the American Speech-Hearing Association (ASHA) have long highlighted the need for working in home language. This takes longer, consumes resources (finance, time) and is more challenging than an English-only approach. Normative data are not available for many populations and the SLT must rely on their training and scientific knowledge. To be truly holistic and achieve the same quality outcomes for our service users, we must endeavour to turn these professional standards into reality. This is no pipe dream. This book is based on best practice that has been successfully delivered in real services in the UK.

## Key learning points

- Bilingualism is the normal language learning pattern for most human beings. Globally, monolinguals are in the minority.

- Bilingualism **never** contributes or causes a speech and language disorder. Professionals should therefore never advise parent(s)/carers to give up the home language to support acquisition of the language of education.

- Bilingualism is **not** a speech and language disorder and should not be listed as a diagnosis.

- Children and young people should always be assessed in **both/all their languages**, and **not compared to monolingual children** for the level of development of each language – bilinguals are not two speakers in one.

- **Normative data based on monolingual children should therefore never be applied to bilingual speakers** as it is an unfair and misleading comparison. This includes age norms, stages of development, percentile ranks, standard scores, and any other measure that is based on monolingual populations. Instead, we must use the bilingual speaker as their own baseline.

- Speech and language therapy services who **deliver assessment, advice, and intervention in both home language and the majority language are more effective** than those that do not. **Intervention in the additional language alone leads to a high risk of home language loss and such a service is inherently discriminatory.**

- **The role of the SLT is to maintain, develop, or restore bilingualism** (Royal College of Speech and Language Therapists, 2019). This includes where the child has started to lose home language skills through attrition. Arguing that the child is now dominant in the mainstream language is not sound, especially when there is still an opportunity to restore bilingualism through use of mother tongue at home. Note that "develop or restore" applies to young bilingual children who have missed the opportunity to acquire their home language due to Language Difficulties. Parent(s)/carers would be encouraged to introduce a home-language policy to encourage home-language *acquisition*. It is not the role of the clinician to *teach* home language or additional languages.

## Identity and ownership of terminology

It is impossible to discuss bilingualism in isolation from culture. Language is the medium by which people construct their identity, their place within their family and within wider society.

Bilingualism does not equate with ethnicity. There are bilingual families who are white and do not suffer the racism and exclusion which often accompanies bilingual speakers who are people of colour. Some languages are regarded as high status and may be regarded as a sign of sophistication. For example, white French-English bilingual speakers living in the UK are unlikely to experience prejudice, since French is regarded as an important modern language, valued in the education system.

For most bilingual families however, their home language is viewed as low status or in a negative light. Bilingualism is often viewed with suspicion by monolingual speakers. Seen as unusual, bilingualism is thought to remove focus from learning spoken and written English and so is damaging to the child. These myths and negative attitudes are a direct result of colonialism and racism within the wider society. Speakers of languages other than English such as those from the Indian sub-continent or Africa will likely have identities linked to their ethnicity. High levels of racial discrimination both historically and currently mean that families may not value their home language, internalising these racist attitudes, or at best conceal or minimise the reporting of the use of their home language.

There are also white families who come from cultures which have experienced discrimination and repression, such as Jewish Yiddish speakers, who are seen as outsiders or "other" from the mainstream monolingual English-speaking community.

It is important to keep the complexity of individual experience in mind when discussing bilingualism and the use of home languages. It is rare for us to share exactly the same experience as our service users. For this reason, it is important to value and respect terminology, language labels, religious beliefs, and cultural practices that are shared during interviews. People have ownership of their own culture and identity, and it is not for professionals (especially monolingual white professionals) to impose their own frameworks onto this complexity.

The following definitions should therefore be viewed through the lens of the individual's lived experience, rather than being seen as absolute definitions. After all, professionals are here to serve the needs of the community rather than the other way around. Unfortunately, the privilege and power associated with being professional may mean that families are pressured into conforming to the wider society expectations.

For bilingual families, the main pressure is to prioritise the mainstream language rather than their home language. The outcome of this is, more often than not, language attrition. This not only threatens the child's ability to speak their home language, but also their ability to understand and construct their own unique identity. As professionals we have responsibilities to ensure that families, children, and young people are encouraged to embrace their unique heritage and home language.

## Bilingualism and multilingualism

"Bilingual" literally means "two tongues." In the UK this is the most frequently used term for people who have some knowledge of two or more languages. For people who speak more than two languages, we can be specific and list the number, such as trilingual, and so on. However, for most international authors, the umbrella term "Multilingual(-ism)" is employed. Other terms have been employed, such as "dual language" (Genesee et al., 2004) and of course "mother tongue." The latter emphasises the fact that women are most frequently the language model for their children, since they undertake the vast majority of the childcare. I favour the terms "home language" and "language of education" as they are transparent and inclusive (see below).

In this book I use "bilingual(-ism)" to encompass children and young people who speak two *or more* languages.

- Many terms are used for speakers of more than one language.
- "Bilingualism" and "multilingualism" are the most frequently encountered.

*Home language, mother tongue, and "our tongue"*

The term "mother tongue" is replaced with "home language," as this acknowledges that there are single parents, adoptive parents, same-sex couples, and gender-diverse parents.

Families tend to use their community language at home and with others from their speech community, so the term seems apt. This contrasts with "additional language," which in the UK and US tends to be the language of education, that is English. It is acknowledged that the situation is not this simple. There are Welsh-language medium schools in Wales, UK, and Gaelic speakers in Scotland.

Many communities simply use terms such as "Apni zaban" (literally, "our tongue") instead of a language label such as "Mirpuri."

- "Home language" is a more inclusive term for the language spoken in the home environment, as well as with extended family and the speech community.

*Mother tongue or mother language*

The United Nations defines mother tongue as the "language usually spoken in the individual's home in his early childhood, although not necessarily used by him at present" (Romaine, 1995, p. 19). As De Luca (2018, p. 161) points out "This . . . has a particular relevance for minority language groups where mother tongue is primarily a spoken medium, often ascribed low status."

International Mother Language Day has been celebrated on the 21st of February each year since 2015, to encourage education for all in their mother tongue. Awareness of the fragility of many mother languages is also an aim of the day. Over 50% of the 7,000 or so languages spoken across the globe are likely to die out within a few generations (UN News, 2015).

Mother tongue is a positive force, with several key benefits in education, leading to better academic results, particularly for girls, and improved literacy and fluency levels In both mother tongue and the majority language (United Nations Special Rapporteur on minority issues, 2017).

*Additional language/Second language*

Technically, "additional language" implies that the speaker is sequentially bilingual (see below). This is the term most frequently used in this book to refer to the language of wider society, the language of education, and of government. In the UK this is English in England and Welsh in Wales. Gaelic is making gains in Scotland (following the Welsh model). Since *most* children and young people in the UK acquire bilingualism in a sequential manner, this terminology usually causes no difficulties.

Other terms are frequently encountered in the literature but are problematic in one way or another. For example, "majority language" may be factually accurate, but can imply to families that this is somehow the "correct" or high-status language, encouraging the family to integrate and abandon the home language. "Language of education" also carries connotations of status and "correctness." Relative language status is important, as negative attitudes toward community languages are common, even amongst speakers of those languages.

For most bilingual speakers in the UK, English is the additional language. English (both spoken and written) is seen as the "default" language. This is because most people speak English and only English. The preponderance of English monolingual speakers makes them believe that bilingualism is unusual (Crystal, 1997). They couldn't be more wrong. If an alien visiting the Earth wished to capture a typical human being, it would not be one of these unusual monolingual speakers! Most of the population of the globe speak one or more additional languages to their home language, to some degree of proficiency. Bilingualism is the norm, and it is important to bear this in mind when counselling bilingual families. Many monolingual professionals imagine that bilingualism is onerous and complex, and should therefore be avoided, especially when the child has a speech, language, or communication need. This could not be further from the truth, and bilingualism has never been found to cause or contribute to a speech or language disorder (Royal College of Speech and Language Therapists, 2019).

- "Additional language(s)" are acquired after the home language in sequential bilingual speakers.
- Most bilingual speakers are from communities where a language is spoken at home and in the community, and the additional language is learnt through attendance in care and education settings.
- Only a relatively small number of bilinguals are simultaneous bilinguals in the UK.
- In the UK, Australia, and US, English is the most commonly encountered additional language, as it is most frequently the language of education, media, and popular entertainment.
- Some communities will have different additional languages, such as English speakers acquiring Welsh in Wales, UK.

## Language

A language is the rule-based use of a symbolic code to forge social links, transmit meaning, and cooperate with others. It is typically transmitted using speech but may be non-verbal using hand and finger signs and facial expression. Semantic meaning is encoded into thematic roles, and then encoded into words and finally a continuous stream of speech (or signs).

Language itself is not the only component of human interaction. Facial expression, social situation, context, past experience of the event or person/people, and cultural knowledge and expectations have a huge influence on the spoken (or signed) message.

People often make the mistake of thinking that language is primarily about sending and receiving messages. Human beings are primarily social beings and use language from the earliest stages of development to form interpersonal bonds. This allows the infant to achieve and survive by being part of a family, extended family, tribe, or community.

Pragmatics, the norms for a situation, and culture play an enormous role in the expectations of play, interaction, and allowable responses. Children who are unfamiliar with Western culture may by surprised or withdrawn in certain situations, since they have no understanding of these alien interactions.

Children and young people with very different life experiences may fail language assessments due to being unfamiliar with the objects, people, and/or activities. Books and interacting with adults may be unusual. For example, Pakistani-heritage children may fail to make eye contact with adults as to make eye contact is seen as rude.

Children may also have different terms or ways of thinking due to language and cultural differences. For example, there are no superlatives (such as "biggest" or "smallest") in Mirpuri.

It is important to note that spoken language does not necessarily have a written form, and literacy is a relatively recent invention. For most of the history of humanity, we have spoken, but not written down our language. Even as more people have become literate, many people around the world have difficulty accessing formal education, especially girls and women. It should not be assumed that anyone can read their spoken language, or even that a written form exists for every language. Some texts such as Arabic and Hebrew are read right-to-left in contrast to English. In highly literate societies, people living in poverty may have limited literacy skills and professionals should default to verbal communication.

- Language is distinct from speech.
- Language is an arbitrary code. Hockett highlighted that, "There is no dependence of the elements of the signal on the nature of the reality to which it refers . . ." (Crystal, 1997, p. 401).
- Language does not necessarily involve speech as humans can encode language using other modalities including sign language, symbol systems and using visual symbols in written language.
- Language is primarily social.
- Language cannot be considered alone. The pragmatic elements are extremely important and are culturally set.
- Children and young people may be unfamiliar with formal language assessment, the use of books, interacting with adults or may fail to recognise the situations used in assessment.

- Children in unfamiliar situations may be silent or fail to answer as completely as those familiar with the testing culture.
- Information leaflets, advice and therapy programmes are often translated in vain, when it would be more cost-effective and more readily available to the family in the form of an audio or video recording of an interpreter.

## Speech

Speech is a code system which facilitates the transmission of language through the air to the listener's ear. Meaning is transposed into phonemes, and these psycholinguistic units then encode meaning into speech acts. **You have never heard or spoken a phoneme.** Phonemes are units of contrast that are encoded into phones. Speech acts are executed by the vocal tract. This results in an airstream being acted upon by articulators and resonant chambers.

Speech is not composed of words. If you hear a language that you do not understand, there are not convenient spaces after each word! It is thought that the largest unit of speech is the syllable. Within the syllable, there are phones. These **phones** (sounds) are transmitted as pressure waves (compressions and rarefactions) through the air.

The listener's ear drum is affected by the sound waves and moves the auditory ossicles (malleus, incus, and stapes). The movement of the auditory ossicles sets up pressure waves in the fluid of the cochlear. This stimulates the hair cells, which in turn send nerve signals to the auditory cortex. The auditory cortex interprets these nerve signals and maps them onto phonemes. The listener then decodes the stream of phonemes into words and back into meaning.

Suprasegmental aspects such as intonation, word tone (for some languages), word stress and voice quality may also form part of the message. These aspects are controlled by vocal pitch and loudness, and so superimposed onto the segments (phones or sounds) of speech.

- Speech is distinct from language.
- Speech is a code which allows verbal speakers to transmit language over a distance.
- Speech in and of itself has no meaning. Only another speaker of that language who has the "map" of contrasts and inventory of phones may decode the speech.
- It is important to consider the speech chain, as children may have difficulties at one or more stage.
- Most speech disorders are **not** physical in nature but are a difficulty in mapping meaning onto a sound code (phonological in nature).

- The speech code for each language may be very different. Bilingual children must therefore learn the mapping (phonological inventory and contrasts mapped to the meaning) for each language.
- Bilingual children may have different phonological processes in each language.

## Codeswitching

Language is also known as a *code*. This is a very apt term, since the words and morphemes we employ for a particular language are arbitrary; that is, they are entirely specific to that language or code, and have no external meaning outside that language. For example, the thing we sit on is a "chair" in English, but /ˈkʊɾ.si/ in Mirpuri.

When a monolingual speaker hears two (or more) bilingual people talking, they may notice that the bilingual conversation has words from two or more languages. Codeswitching, literally changing from one language or code to another, is a very common and normal phenomenon. This seems to happen randomly to the untrained ear, and for this reason is sometimes referred to as *code mixing*. I dislike this term since codeswitching is rule-bound and not merely a jumbled "mix" of words from the speaker's languages! As we will see, this has important implications for the assessment of bilingual children's language skills. Codeswitching may also occur bimodally (spoken and signed languages) in exactly the same way as two spoken languages.

*Code, code switching, or codeswitching*

A code is a language. A switch is a change from one language to another (or back again). Each language has a syntactic framework, which orders how content (lexical items) are organised.

A bilingual person may change or switch their languages in two ways:

1.  Utterance in language 1 followed by utterance in language 2
    For example, "Lovely to see you, Dieter! **Wie geht es dir?**" *(How going is dative case + singular?)*
    (L1 = English/**L2 = German**)

    This is known as **intersentential** codeswitching
    (**between** *sentences change of language*)
2.  A "bilingual utterance" where elements are taken from both languages
    For example, "**Girl chair** aper beh-ti vi" *(girl chair on sit-ing + female is + female)*

In this example, the speaker has retained the Mirpuri phrase order and morphology; compare it with the monolingual Mirpuri utterance:

"kuri kursi aper beh-ti vi" *(girl chair on sit-ing + female is + female)*

The content words (nouns and verbs) are often drawn from one language (in this case, English), while the frame is still recognisably Mirpuri.

This is known as *intrasentential codeswitching*

(*within* sentence change of language)

Languages don't contribute equally to a bilingual utterance. Usually, one language sets the syntactic structure (frame), while content words (nouns and verbs) are drawn from the other language (See Myers-Scotton, 2002 for an in-depth model of intrasentential codeswitching). The child or young person views the words as synonyms rather than a change of language.

Codeswitching is clinically relevant as children's longest and most complex utterances are those containing codeswitching (Pert & Letts, 2003). Codeswitching also increases with age, showing this is a sign of linguistic sophistication and not, as previous observers have posited, a sign of confusion. The fact that children produce their "best" utterances when they have access to both languages makes perfect sense. If a child is forced by the pragmatic situation to use only one of their languages, then they are highly restricted. Only "bilingual utterances," where the child is able to draw on their full linguistic knowledge, provide us with an insight into their expressive language capabilities. This is another reason why additional language–only assessment is a poor substitute for working alongside an interpreter.

Codeswitching may be viewed in a negative light by both monolingual speakers and bilingual speakers. This is true even of communities who routinely use a mixed code. Speakers will often deny that they could switch as they perceive codeswitched utterances to be inferior to monolingual utterances (Dewaele & Wei, 2014). This leads to contradictory behaviour to that reported. Parents of bilingual children will often insist that they use one language per parent or carer, the "one-person one language" approach. Despite this, bilingual people cannot help but codeswitch. Goodz (1989, p. 25) found that "a large proportion of parents, even those firmly committed to maintaining a strict separation of language by parent, model linguistically mixed utterances for their children." This shows how unconscious and automatic codeswitching is, and how futile it is to try and control what is a normal and frequent behaviour of almost all bilingual speakers.

• Codeswitching is the use of two (or more languages) in a conversation, and sometimes in a single spoken sentence or bilingual utterance.

- Codeswitching is normal and frequently encountered in bilingual-to-bilingual conversations.
- Codeswitching is a sign of linguistic sophistication, not of confusion.
- Avoiding codeswitching is not a desirable aim and will not contribute to the care of typically developing bilingual children, or those with a Speech Sound Disorder or language disorder.
- Codeswitched "bilingual utterances" are the best measure of a bilingual child's expressive language.

## Developmental Language Disorder (DLD) versus the defunct "language delay" diagnostic label

"Language delay" or "delayed language skills" are diagnostic labels that have been used for many years by SLTs. The terms are misleading and confusing. The terms were often used as justification for not intervening immediately. Children were often discharged or "monitored," and so the diagnostic labels became a way for SLTs to manage busy caseloads. The terms suggest that the child or young person will "catch up," although the evidence shows that this is unlikely after the age of 5 years.

Some SLTs, confused by the diagnostic labels, have suggested that "delayed language" becomes "disordered language" after some arbitrary date. Yet others think that there is some qualitative difference between the expression of children with delayed language versus those with disordered language. I was taught (incorrectly) that children with disordered language will have phrase or word-order errors, and other unusual features, whereas children with delayed language will simply produce language that is akin to the language output of younger children. The evidence base does not support this.

The situation is even muddier when learning difficulties are present. SLTs often ceased treatment or denied access to specialist or intensive resources such as language provisions based on the false assumption that children and young people with learning difficulties had "language in line with their learning" and therefore would not benefit from this provision. Only those children with "spikey profiles" would be eligible. A similar argument was made for those children living in poverty. That somehow, such children were "delayed" and would inevitably catch up. Again, the evidence base does not support this (Bishop et al., 2016).

For bilingual children, similar claims have been made, with "delayed language" applied to children exclusively from the monolingual mainstream viewpoint. To assess only in the mainstream language will always make bilingual children appear behind compared to their monolingual peers. It obviously takes more processing of input language data and acquisition time to acquire two or more languages compared to one. The use of "delay" also ignores the child's home-language skills. The term "delayed language" should there-fore never be applied to bilingual children (Hegde & Maul, 2006). Instead use "Language Difficulties" or "Speech, Language, and Communication Needs" (SLCN) (below the age of 5) and "Developmental Language Disorder"/"Language Disorder associated with X" (where X is any recognised biomedical condition) (after the age of 5, or earlier if the Language Difficulty is likely to persist beyond 5 years of age). Please see Bishop et al. (2016, 2017); and Ebbels (2020) for a thorough exploration of the evidence and use of the new terminology.

## Language acquisition in bilingual children

Bilingualism is often considered by describing *when* a child acquires their languages. Either one after the other – sequential bilingualism, or at the same time – simultaneous bilingual-ism. From a speech and language therapy perspective, both types are valid and will not usually cause any difficulties for the child.

Raising a child in a bilingual environment does not cause language disorder, nor does it aggravate existing difficulties, such as Language Disorder (Korkman et al., 2012).

- Typical bilingual/multilingual language acquisition never causes or contributes to a speech, language, or communication disorder.
- Many terms and perspectives on typical language acquisition exist. It is not the remit of this book to review typical bilingual language acquisition.

## One Person One Language approach (OPOL)

This approach arises from research into language acquisition, where linguists sought to track where children were exposed to a particular lexical item label. By asking the par-ents to use one language each, the child's language acquisition in each language could be monitored.

There was also a myth that children were "confused" by hearing two or more languages in the home. The evidence for this was codeswitched utterances (bilingual utterances). We now know that codeswitching is normal, and a sign of linguistic sophistication. We also know that parents, even those purportedly using a one-person one-language approach, codeswitch at times (Goodz, 1989). So, is there any clinical merit in recommending this approach to parents and carers?

For most families, the adults will codeswitch as part of normal bilingual conversation and recommending the approach may be unrealistic. For single parent families, the approach is just not possible.

There are instances where the approach may be practical and desirable. These families are relatively rare and tend to be elite, highly educated families. In order for a child to receive sufficient exposure to two (or more) language, families may use this approach. However, two parents or carers need to ensure that they deliver approximately the same amount of childcare, or the language of the parent with least contact is unlikely to be successfully acquired. Therefore, the approach requires employment with flexible working patterns across the couple. For most children and young people, this type of arrangement is not possible. Byers-Heinlein and Lew-Williams (2013, p. 4) highlight that, although some children may acquire two languages successfully, others do not, and that the one-person one-language approach is "neither *necessary* nor *sufficient* for successful bilingual acquisition."

- The OPOL approach will not prevent a child from confusing languages, because children cope exceeding well with two or more languages, even if they have a language disorder.
- The OPOL approach seeks to keep the two languages separate, and this is not how typical bilingual individuals use their languages. Codeswitching is normal and frequently encountered. Parents/carers codeswitch frequently, often without realising that they are doing it.
- The OPOL approach requires roughly even allocation of childcare to ensure sufficient language exposure time (Baker, 2000a), and only families with flexible working arrangements are able to achieve this. For these families, the OPOL approach may ensure that the child acquires both languages simultaneously.

## Potential bilingual/monolingual in a Language Other Than English (LOTE)

Many children are referred to as "bilingual" or "multilingual" simply because they don't speak the majority language. This is inaccurate. Young children, or those who have not yet commenced additional language acquisition, are *potentially bilingual* or *monolingual in a language other than X* (where X is typically English or Welsh). For the majority of children in the UK, this applies to children who have not yet started education (or do not attend a care setting), or those newly arrived in the country.

Some children within this group will have encountered English via television programmes, neighbours, shopping with parents, and other interactions, and they may have begun to acquire receptive bilingualism. That is, they have the ability to understand an additional language, but cannot yet use it functionally.

- Children labelled "bilingual" or "multilingual" may actually be **potentially bilingual** if they have yet to start acquiring an additional language, or **receptively bilingual** if they only have (developing) verbal comprehension skills.

## Language acquisition versus formal language learning

Young children do not have lessons in language instruction. Rather, they acquire the language through exposure to a language or languages and use language to interact with their carers, family, and friends.

In contrast, learning a "foreign language" is often an academic pursuit, with lessons, textbooks, and audio recordings to listen to and imitate.

The main differences are

- Age of exposure
- Pragmatic acquisition versus conscious learning
- Usage in everyday life/activities

It has been hotly debated in the literature as to both how children acquire language and at what age they cease to have the skill to acquire a language rather than learn it formally.

Many English monolingual speakers have encountered some foreign language formal teaching, typically learning European languages such as French or German, but do not consider themselves bilingual as they do not use the language on a daily or regular basis or may not have progressed beyond rote learning of useful phrases with which to order food and drink, book train tickets or ask for directions.

## Sequential bilingualism

This is when a child learns their home language, followed an additional language. The additional language is typically the language of education, and it is when a child enters a care or educational setting that they are exposed to the additional language and expected to acquire that language.

This is the most frequently encountered route to bilingualism in the UK.

## Simultaneous bilingualism

This is when a child is exposed to two (or more) languages at the same time. This "bilingualism as a home language" approach depends on the child having sufficient exposure to the languages and opportunities to use both languages.

## Heritage language

The term *heritage language* is used in this book. For example, Pakistani-heritage languages include Mirpuri, Punjabi, and Urdu. Montrul (2016, p. 2) defines heritage-language speakers as "child and adult members of a linguistic minority who grow up exposed to their home language – the heritage language – and the majority official language spoken and used in the broader speech community."

Heritage-language speakers are the most frequently encountered populations in the UK. This is linked with a history of immigration and Empire.

It is important to establish the precise language or languages spoken by a person or family. Families may report the most well-known language label, usually that of the most high-status variant rather than an accurate one (See Accent and Dialect).

- Heritage languages are typically, but not always associated with an immigrant community that have established a community in another country.
- For established communities, most speakers will acquire the heritage language as their home language, with many speakers also acquiring the mainstream language.
- Most speakers after the first generation will be citizens of the country the original immigrants moved to. For example, there are established Pakistani- and Bangladeshi-heritage communities in the UK with several generations of British Asian people.

- It is not possible to assume that a person from a particular cultural heritage will automatically speak the heritage language. Ethnicity does not correlate with bilingualism! For example, British Asian people may only speak English; or speak a home language/ languages and English.
- Some families may have become monolingual English speakers but choose to rediscover their bilingual heritage. For example, a British Asian couple who are monolingual English speakers may learn Urdu and then raise their children to speak English and Urdu.

## High-status and low-status languages

All languages are equally complex and valid. It is nonsense to claim that one language is superior to another. However, human beings are emotive creatures, and attach value or stigma to particular languages. More benign examples of this are impressions of a language. Many English speakers claim that French is "romantic," German is "harsh," and US accents are "cool." Rather than properties of the languages themselves, these are obviously perceptions and (illogical) cultural stereotypes of the nations and their speakers, and not of the phonology, syntax, grammar, and morphology!

More importantly, status can affect whether a language lives or dies. Negative attitudes to a language can see rapid decline in its use, until it is lost completely. The status of a language, that is, how much it is valued by others and even the speakers of the language themselves, is dependent on a wide range of social, societal, and historic factors. English-speaking societies including the UK, Australia, and US have a long history of oppressing native languages and supplanting them with English. This is a form of cultural occupation that matches the physical occupation of the territory.

Languages linked to education and subsequent success in employment are therefore often valued more than home languages. If a home language or heritage language is in contact with a high-status language, there is a high risk that the speaker will speak less and less of home language until it is lost. This is termed *language loss*.

Languages can change status over time, illustrating that status is not an intrinsic and independent feature of a language, but rather the cultural and societal perception of that language. An example of this is Welsh. Cymraeg (or "Welsh") is one of the oldest languages in Europe and was spoken by over 90% of the community in Wales at the end of the 19th century. Successive interventions by the English government, including

English education for Welsh monolingual speakers, led to a dramatic decline in Welsh. English-language education for Welsh speaking children has been described as part of an attitude of "the superiority of English culture, and involved neglect of the Welsh language and culture, [and] epitomizes the hallmark of an internal colonial model" (Hetcher, 1975 in Evans, 1993). It was the efforts of the Welsh people that saved the language from the brink of extinction. Today, almost a third of the population speak Welsh, with a target of a million speakers by 2050 (Llywodraeth Cymru – Welsh Government, 2017). Welsh language schools, media, and politics are all part of Welsh culture. Welsh is now a high-status language, growing in speakers after many decades of being a low-status, disappearing language. This reversal of fortunes illustrates that languages need community support to thrive.

- Language status tends to be linked with perceptions of social and educational prestige and success.
- Low-status language speakers may not value their home language.
- The status of a language may change over time.
- A high-status language is likely to replace a low-status language within a speaker, family, or community unless professions highlight the advantages of home languages.

## The impact of language status on the individual and bilingual family

Parents and carers want the best educational outcomes for their children. This can affect the attitude to home language use versus the use of the language of education in the home environment. This is a complex issue and parents' beliefs need to be discussed and objective information provided.

Parents may believe that forgoing bilingualism and speaking only the language of education (typically English) will enhance their child's educational success. This has surface validity, but there may be severe problems with this in practice. For example, if the parents do not have excellent English language skills themselves, children will receive a poor language model for their language acquisition. Parents may be surprised that speaking mainly or only the language of education will lead to monolingualism. Unintended consequences, such as not being able to speak to relatives and the community, and failure to understand their culture may therefore be unexpected outcomes for the child.

Children and young people may suffer isolation from their parent(s) and extended family if they do not have access to their home language. Home language is also how culture and concepts within that culture are transmitted. A loss of identity and ability to seek support may lead to poor mental health.

- The language of education (English, Welsh) confers high status.
- Parents and carers may feel pressure to abandon their home language and use the language of education.
- Abandonment of the home language may lead to poor language acquisition and social and cultural isolation for the child or young person.
- Mental health is at risk if a child or young person cannot communicate with their family, extended family, and wider community.

## Pre-literate language versus illiteracy

Language is spoken (or signed for sign languages). Before the discovery of writing, including alphabetic system, and syllabary written symbol systems, spoken language had existed for millennia. Written language is a relatively new invention compared to spoken language. Writing systems are thought to have evolved independently in different cultures at least four times, with the oldest writing system originating in Mesopotamia almost 5,500 years ago (Clayton, 2019).

This is easily forgotten in the highly literate world of the west. Text and speech seem completely interchangeable. Literacy rates are uneven across the globe due to economic, social, and political factors. Literacy rates continue to rise, with the youth population (15–24 years) at 91% and adult population (25–64 years) at 86%. This still leaves 609 million people illiterate (UNESCO Institute for Statistics, 2017).

It is important to note that illiteracy is more common in girls and women due to exclusion from education, either by policy, tradition or demands on females to act as carers. Many countries only have basic education and/or no universal free education system. Many speakers will not, therefore be able to read the text for their language.

Some languages have no written form for the spoken language. These languages are termed preliterate. An example is Mirpuri. It is therefore not possible to write this language down, other than by using the International Phonetic Alphabet (IPA), and this is not retrievable by non-specialists. Speakers of this language can rarely read the related but distinct languages Punjabi or Urdu, which do have written forms, and if they can, are likely to be educated to a level where they have had the opportunity to learn spoken and written English.

For SLTs, this should inform all the work we do. Verbal communication is superior when providing information than written. Most adults are too embarrassed to say that they cannot read and write, or that their language has no written form.

Even for English monolingual speakers, many service users live in poverty and may have had poor experiences in education themselves. The default should therefore be spoken communication.

- Many parent(s) and carers have poor literacy/no literacy skills.
- Some languages have no written form.
- Even if there is a written form, many people will not be able to read their own language.
- Translation of written materials into home language are likely to be a "tick box" exercise.
- Appointment letters/texts, advice leaflets, reports, and therapy programmes are best presented in the family's home language. This may be achieved by the parent(s)/carer recording you/an interpreter reading out the relevant information, or by making videos and sending a link for families to view.

## Accent and dialect

It may seem odd to discuss accent and dialect in the context of bilingualism. The UK is renowned for having different ways of speaking across the regions, with a person from Yorkshire sounding different in their vowel system, use of glottal stops, and other minor phonetic differences compared to a "standard English" speaker. Simply ask how people pronounce the baked treat with cream and jam ("scone") and sit back as the heated debate between different speakers erupts!

Different dialects are characterised by some changes in lexical item, such as what people call a small individual serving of bread: bread roll, cob, bun, stottie cake, or barm cake, to name but a few (YouGov, 2018).

Although there is no strict differential between "accent" and "dialect," most observers associate accent with speech sound differences, and dialect with lexical and/or grammatical differences. With mass media including film, television, and radio, as well as on-demand services online, the UK is expected to experience a convergence of language with regional differences slowly eroding over the next half century (Burridge & Blaxter, 2020).

English regional accents/dialects may puzzle foreign visitors who have only ever encountered "standard English" (spoken in the southeast of England, associated with prestige and power of Parliament, royalty, and the BBC). However, to most people, speakers are perfectly intelligible, and accent and dialect are noted as signs of social class, geography of childhood upbringing, and a feature of (mainly) northern English. There are rarely changes in syntax or grammar, and breakdown in understanding rarely occurs.

For other languages, what a speaker may refer to as a "dialect," "slang," or "accent" may in fact be a completely separate language that is not mutually intelligible. The motivations for describing the languages as "dialects" (or similar) may be due to an overlap of lexical items, similar/related language origins, and concepts of national identity.

For example, Mirpuri, Punjabi, and Urdu are not fully mutually intelligible. They share almost 79% of the same vocabulary and word/phrase order, and yet have very different verb phrases and morphology. Adults cannot usually understand everything that is said (unless fluent in all three languages), and children would certainly not understand instructions if the wrong "variant" were used by an adult.

- Research the language spoken in your local catchment area, using local government statistics and/or an audit of your referrals and caseload from the previous year.
- Offer a choice of languages that you know are spoken in your catchment area. For example, ask a Pakistani-heritage family, "Do you speak Mirpuri, Punjabi, or Urdu?" rather than "Which language do you speak?"
- All languages have a high-status variant and a low-status variant. Ensure that you have the correct interpreter for the dialect spoken. Families will not always feel able to object if a high-status variant speaker is present due to issues of respect, so it is your role to check this carefully.
- Children may fail assessments if the wrong language or dialect is employed.
- "Dialects"/"Accents" should be considered separate languages.

## The evolution of terminology and speaker's preferences

Just as in many other scientific and social arenas, the terminology relating to bilingualism and speech and language disorders is subject to change. This change often reflects a scientific insight, a need to standardise definitions, or the rise of a particular term over another. Recent examples include the revision of Specific Language Impairment (SLI) to

Developmental Language Disorder (DLD), Language Delay being abandoned (Bishop et al., 2016, 2017), and Multilingualism versus Bilingualism.

The SLT must commit to a lifelong-learning culture and remain up-to-date with the ever-evolving terminology.

Similarly, children and families who access services may perceive themselves and their bilingualism in many different ways. Terminology used by a parent, carer, or children and young people themselves may closely align with ties to family, culture, and identity. As such, these terms should always be respected. As we will see later, there can be clashes between a family's culture and that of professionals. Respectful navigation of these differences is one of the most important aspects of delivering assessment and care. Professionals need not, and should not, insist that their terminology, perspective, and beliefs supersede those of the people they are supposed to care for and serve. Only when a child or young person is in danger of neglect or abuse should this principle be displaced.

## Language attrition

Language attrition is when a speaker's first language undergoes disintegration due to contact with a second language (Seliger & Vago, 1991).

This is important for several reasons. Firstly, typically developing children are likely to lose their home language if they are not encouraged to use it daily at home. Secondly, we need to consider that bilingual children may become more successful additional language learners if they are supported in their home language. This may seem counter-intuitive at first glance. One would anticipate that if a child received intervention in home language, it would be that language which develops. However, this is to overlook cross-linguistic transfer. Languages are all symbolic systems that encode ideas, concepts and intentions as messages encoding into speech (or signs). Children may learn a concept or idea in one language, and although direct learning will not be the same in the additional language (due to surface difference such as phrase order and morphological encoding), the child will not have to learn the same concepts again. Rather, the child only needs to understand that there are two labels or ways or expressing that concept or idea.

## Cross-linguistic transfer

Children with two or more languages can differentiate between those languages from an early age. However, unlike monolingual children, bilingual children can draw on knowledge from both languages. Observations of application of knowledge of one language to another has been observed in bilingual children. Nicoladis (2006, p. 25) provides examples of French-English phrase which are structured as if they are French utterances. For example, "a monkey purple," where a French phrase order has been employed for an English utterance. If following the English phrase order, where adjectives precede the head noun, the phrase would be "a purple monkey." Although there are many possible explanations for these phenomena, it is unsurprising that children use the full breadth of their language knowledge and experiment with different formulations. It does seem that children have at least some transfer between their languages, especially if two of their languages share similarities.

If children and young people can transfer language learning gains in one language to the other, why not simply use the mainstream or majority language for intervention (such as English)? This would usually be easier for professionals and be lower in cost due to the fact that an interpreter would not be required and materials in other languages produced.

The problem with the above approach is that if children prefer one language over another, they are likely to lose the less favoured language rather than develop both languages. Language loss rather than language addition is especially notable where the status of one language is lower than the other. For the SLT, this means that intervention in a high-status language such as English is likely to result in complete loss of the home language. This is why relying on cross-linguistic effects is not possible when delivering language therapy.

## Populations and terminology

Not all bilingual people are from a non-white background. However, in the UK, and around the world, a significant number of families will speak a language other than English and are also from a community of non-white people. "White" is a UK government census term, and I am using "non-white" not to exclude people or be offensive, but as a prelude to a discussion about which terms are applied and which terms are acceptable to these communities.

Terminology for populations have changed over the years in response to changing fashions, recognition of different political and social changes and increasing sensitivity to the right of a community to define themselves.

In the literature you may encounter many different terms, including "ethnic minority," "minority ethnic," "Black, Asian, and Minority Ethnic" (often as the acronym BAME), and "People of Colour" (or "People of Color" in the US).

It is my view that communities should choose their own terminology. For a person outside that community to apply a label, especially one that is rejected by that community, is an example of racism.

When these labels are explored, they are often found wanting. They fail to identify a person within their community accurately, often bracketing together many disparate groups, and often fail to encapsulate a person's own experience of their ethnicity. For example, Bhopal (2004, p. 441) illustrates the shortcomings of the term "Asian," which in the UK is often understood to refer to "persons whose ancestry is from the Indian subcontinent," whereas in the US this term "was interpreted as far Eastern Asian populations."

BAME has been criticised for being too vague. Choudrey (2022, p. 28) states that "One of the criticisms is how often and how easily Black is conflated with BAME. Statistics that speak for BAME populations sometimes don't include any Black communities."

The UK government employs a set of 19 ethnic groups, included under five main headings:

- Asian or Asian British
  - Indian
  - Pakistani
  - Bangladeshi
  - Chinese
  - Any other Asian background
- Black, Black British, Caribbean, or African
  - Caribbean
  - African
  - Any other Black, Black British, or Caribbean background
- Mixed or multiple ethnic groups
  - White and Black Caribbean
  - White and Black African
  - White and Asian
  - Any other Mixed or multiple ethnic background
- White
  - English, Welsh, Scottish, Northern Irish, or British
  - Irish
  - Gypsy or Irish Traveller

- Roma
  - Any other White background
- Other ethnic group
  - Arab
  - Any other ethnic group

(ONS, 2022)

Consensus is lacking in this area, and some individuals or communities may object to analysis by ethnicity in principle. However, professionals and researchers must use some terms so that communities are not excluded from reports, research, and service planning which aim to serve these populations.

For services and individual practitioners, the most pragmatic and easy answer is to directly ask the family, "What do you consider your ethnicity to be?" rather than present a pre-devised tick-box menu of options. Services and researchers may wish to audit such responses to identify recurring themes in the terminology provided and involve members of the community to devise a co-produced set of terms.

### People who are refugees and people seeking asylum

A person who is a refugee is someone who has been forced to flee their own country because their safety and life is put at risk. This may be because of conflict, war or because their own government cannot, or will not protect them from danger (Amnesty International, 2022).

When people reach another country, they are legally entitled to request sanctuary. A person seeking asylum is therefore someone who is waiting for a decision to be processed on their application for asylum in a country of safety (UNHCR, 2021).

People seeking asylum are extremely vulnerable. Asylum claims may take many months or even years to process in the UK (Hewett, 2021). Often traumatised by what they have witnessed and/or experienced, they fear that they may be deported back to the country they have fled. People seeking asylum are often wary of health providers as they "fear . . . that (they) may be government informers on people without legal settlement" (Mudyarabikwa et al., 2021, p. 200).

When working with people seeking asylum, it is especially important to ensure that interpreters are aware of their professional duty towards confidentiality. The available pool of interpreters for a particular language community may be very small, and the interpreter may even be known to the family.

*Immigrants and migrants*

People who are migrants are those who do not meet the legal definition of a refugee but have left their home country. This may be for study, for work, to be with family members, or for another reason. Amnesty International (2022) highlights that people who are migrants may also fear persecution or danger to their person.

# References

Amnesty International. (2022). *Refugees, asylum-seekers and migrants*. Retrieved March 13, 2022, from www.amnesty.org/en/what-we-do/refugees-asylum-seekers-and-migrants

Baker, C. (2000a). *A parents' and teachers' guide to bilingualism*. Multilingual Matters Ltd.

Baker, C. (2000b). *The care and education of young bilinguals: An introduction for professionals*. Multilingual Matters.

Bhopal, R. (2004). Glossary of terms relating to ethnicity and race: For reflection and debate. *Journal of Epidemiology and Community Health, 58*, 441–445. http://doi.org/10.1136/jech.2003.013466.

Bishop, D. V. M., Snowling, M. J., Thompson, P. A., & Greenhalgh, T. (2017). Phase 2 of CATALISE: A multinational and multidisciplinary Delphi consensus study of problems with language development: Terminology. *Journal of Child Psychology and Psychiatry, 58*, 1068–1080. https://doi.org/10.1111/jcpp.12721.

Bishop, D. V. M., Snowling, M. J., Thompson, P. A., Greenhalgh, T., & Consortium, C. (2016). CATALISE: A multinational and multidisciplinary Delphi consensus study. Identifying language impairments in children. *PLoS One, 11*, e0158753. https://doi.org/10.1371/journal.pone.0158753

Burridge, J., & Blaxter, T. (2020). Using spatial patterns of English folk speech to infer the universality class of linguistic copying. *Physical Review Research, 2*, 43053. https://doi.org/10.1103/PhysRevResearch.2.043053

Byers-Heinlein, K., & Lew-Williams, C. (2013). Bilingualism in the early years: What the science says. *LEARNing Landscapes, 7*, 95–112. https://doi.org/10.36510/learnland.v7i1.632

Choudrey, S. (2022). *Supporting trans people of colour*. Jessica Kingsley.

Clayton, E. (2019). *A history of writing: where did writing begin?* British Library. www.bl.uk/history-of-writing/articles/where-did-writing-begin#

Crystal, D. (1997). *The Cambridge encyclopedia of language* (2nd ed.). Cambridge University Press.

Cunningham-Andersson, U., & Andersson, S. (2004). *Growing up with two languages: a practical guide* (2nd ed.). Routledge.

De Luca, C. (2018). Mother tongue as a universal human right. *International Journal of Speech Language Pathology, 20*(1), 161–165. https://doi.org/10.1080/17549507.2017.1392606.

Dewaele, J. M., & Wei, J. M. (2014). Attitudes towards code-switching among adult mono- and multilingual language users. *Journal of Multilingual and Multicultural Development*. https://doi.org/10.1080/01434632.2013.859687.

Ebbels, S. (2020, November 19). *DLD – when is a diagnosis appropriate?* YouTube: Royal College of Speech and Language Therapists. www.youtube.com/watch?v=TOPiu-o9fJO.

Evans, W. G. (1993). The bilingual difficulty – HMI and the Welsh Language in the Victorian age. *Welsh History Review, 16*(4), 494–513.

Genesee, F., Paradis, J., & Crago, M. B. (2004). *Dual language development & disorders: A handbook on bilingualism and second language learning* (Vol. 11). Paul H. Brookes Publishing Company.

Goodz, N. S. (1989). Parental language mixing in bilingual families. *Infant Mental Health Journal, 10*(1), 25–44. https://doi.org/10.1002/1097-0355(198921)10:1%3C25::AID-IMHJ2280100104%3E3.0.CO;2-R

Hegde, M. N., & Maul, C. A. (2006). *Language disorders in children: An evidence-based approach to assessment and treatment*. Pearson.

Hewett, A. (2021). *Living in Limbo: A decade of delays in the UK asylum system*. Refugee Council. https://media.refugeecouncil.org.uk/wp-content/uploads/2021/07/01191305/Living-in-Limbo-A-decade-of-delays-in-the-UK-Asylum-system-July-2021.pdf

Korkman, M., Stenroos, M., Mickos, A., Westman, M., Ekholm, P., & Byring, R. (2012). Does simultaneous bilingualism aggravate children's specific language problems? *Acta Paediatrica, 101*(9), 946–952. https://doi.org/10.1111/j.1651-2227.2012.02733.x.

Llywodraeth Cymru – Welsh Government. (2017). *Cymraeg 2050: A million Welsh speakers*. Welsh Language Division. https://www.gov.wales/sites/default/files/publications/2018-12/cymraeg-2050-welsh-language-strategy.pdf

Montrul, S. (2016). *The acquisition of heritage languages*. Cambridge University Press.

Moore, I., Bitchell, L., & Lord, R. (2020). *The health & care professions council equality, diversity and inclusion data 2020 report*. Health and Care Professions Council. Retrieved July 27, 2021, from www.hcpc-uk.org/globalassets/about-us/edi/hcpc-equality-diversity-and-inclusion-data-2020-report.pdf?v=637395820190000000

Mudyarabikwa, O., Regmi, K., Ouillon, S., & Simmonds, R. (2021). Refugee and immigrant community health champions: A qualitative study of perceived barriers to service access and Utilisation of the National Health Service (NHS) in the West Midlands, UK. *Journal of Immigrant and Minority Health*, *24*, 199–206. https://doi.org/10.1007/s10903-021-01233-4

Myers-Scotton, C. (2002). *Contact linguistics: Bilingual encounters and grammatical outcomes*. Oxford University Press.

Myers-Scotton, C. (2005). *Multiple voices: An introduction to bilingualism*. Blackwell Publishing.

Nicoladis, E. (2006). Cross-linguistic transfer in adjective – noun strings by preschool bilingual children. *Bilingualism (Cambridge, England)*, *9*, 15–32. https://doi.org/10.1017/S136672890500235X

Office for National Statistics (ONS). (2022). *List of ethnic groups*. UK Government. Retrieved February 19, 2022, from www.ethnicity-facts-figures.service.gov.uk/style-guide/ethnic-groups

Pert, S., & Letts, C. (2003). Developing an expressive language assessment for children in Rochdale with a Pakistani heritage background. [(34 ref)]. *Child Language Teaching & Therapy*, *19*(3), 267–289. https://doi.org/10.1191%2F0265659003ct255oa.

Romaine, S. (1995). *Bilingualism*. Blackwell Publishing.

Royal College of Speech and Language Therapists. (2019). *Clinical guidelines: Bilingualism*. RCSLT. www.rcslt.org/members/clinical-guidance/bilingualism

Seliger, H. W., & Vago, R. M. (1991). The study of first language attrition: An overview. In H. W. Seliger & R. M. Vago (Eds.), *First language attrition*. Cambridge University Press.

UN News. (2015, February 21). *On mother language day, UN spotlights role of native tongue in education*. https://www.news.un.org/en/story/2015/02/491672-mother-language-day-un-spotlights-role-native-tongue-education

UNESCO Institute for Statistics. (2017, September). *Literacy rates continue to rise from one generation to the next*. Fact Sheet No. 45. http://www.uis.unesco.org/sites/default/files/documents/fs45-literacy-rates-continue-rise-generation-to-next-en-2017_0.pdf

UNHCR UK. (2021). *Asylum-seekers*. Retrieved March 13, 2022, from www.unhcr.org/uk/asylum-seekers.html

United Nations Special Rapporteur on Minority Issues. (2017). *Language rights of linguistic minorities: A practical guide for implementation*. www.ohchr.org/sites/default/files/Documents/Issues/Minorities/SR/LanguageRightsLinguisticMinorities_EN.pdf

YouGov. (2018). *Cobs, buns, baps or barm cakes: What do people call bread rolls?* https://www.yougov.co.uk/topics/food/articles-reports/2018/07/20/cobs-buns-baps-or-barm-cakes-what-do-people-call-b

# DIFFERENTIATING LANGUAGE DISORDER FROM LANGUAGE DIFFERENCE

DOI: 10.4324/9781003125563-3

## Differentiating language disorder from language difference

It is not the role of the SLT to facilitate additional language learning in a child who has already acquired a home language. Similarly, a child acquiring two or more languages in the home will not require speech and language therapy if they are not experiencing difficulties (RCSLT, 2022).

This is because the child who has "cracked the code" of language clearly has the skills to acquire verbal language. This is in contrast with children presenting with language disorder. Such children may have difficulties with short-term memory, segmenting streams of speech into individual lexical items, and associating words with objects, actions, and concepts that they observe in the real world.

So why might a professional be concerned about the English skills of a child who speaks a home language perfectly well? This is the error of assuming that a bilingual child is two speakers in one. That is, that they should have acquired the same speech and language skills as their monolingual peers. Since children who are exposed to home language are then expected to acquire an additional language on school entry, they will clearly take longer to master both languages. This does not make children "language delayed." Rather they have a typical bilingual language acquisition profile. Comparing bilingual children with monolingual children who have only ever heard one language code is clearly an unfair comparison. This means that the use of any mainstream language standardised normative data (including age equivalents, standard scores, percentile ranks, age norms, stages, and any other measure based on monolingual speech and language acquisition) should never be applied to bilingual children. To do so is to directly compare a bilingual child with a monolingual child. Such children have had completely different experiences with the languages being assessed.

**How then, do we assess bilingual children to see if they have difficulty acquiring speech and/or language in any of their languages?**

If a child has a language disorder, or Speech Sound Disorder, these difficulties will be evident in both/all the languages that they hear or speak. This is because the processes involved in mapping language are affected by a central deficit or deficits. It is therefore **not possible for a child who speaks one language perfectly well to have a language disorder in their other language.** If a child only has difficulties in the additional language, then this will be due to lack of exposure or unrealistic expectations of adults on how quickly the language may be acquired. Children require many years to acquire conversational skills, and many more still to think and problem solve in an additional language. The medium to long-term benefits of bilingualism outweigh this initial phase as the child is acquiring two languages and understanding of two cultures. There is research evidence that being bilingual brings increased employment opportunities as well as cognitive advantages.

For young children in the early stages of language acquisition, it may be that on entry to nursery or school that they have little or no language of education. This is not a disorder, and the outcome for children who speak a home language is excellent provided that they are allowed to develop their additional language skills on top of the firm foundation of their home language.

Mistakes are made by well-meaning but misguided professionals who recommend giving up the home language in order to facilitate faster acquisition of the additional language of school. This will lead to language loss of the home language. This is not only a disadvantage linguistically, but also isolates the child from their culture, their extended family, their community and ultimately their sense of identity. We must therefore consider that only negative mental health outcomes are possible when the home language is abandoned. The loss of their home language and cultural identity is one of the main reasons why professionals should never recommend that families abandon the home language in favour of an additional language such as English.

Families who speak home language may have internalised the racist message that their home language and culture are not as valuable as the language and culture of education. This is unsurprising, when languages such as English are promoted as the route to success in education and employment. Furthermore, high-status languages such as English will be encountered by children and young people in pop music, computer games, the Internet, movies, and other cultural activities with high social status and value. Many parents will therefore blame any speech and Language Difficulties on bilingualism itself. This negative view of home language use must be strongly challenged by the multidisciplinary team, including the SLT. Education for parent groups and education staff is crucial to ensure that there is the consistent message that home language is valuable and will not interfere with additional language learning.

## Can children only have problems learning the additional language?

If children have acquired their home language, then they have demonstrated that they have all the appropriate abilities to construct a language from the language input they hear around them. Such an individual cannot possibly have a language disorder.

Other children will have two or more language as their home language. That is, bilingualism as a first language. Such children have access to both/all their languages and even young children do not have difficulties managing the task of switching between languages, producing bilingual utterances with content words from any of their languages, and simultaneously acquiring two or more languages.

Difficulties learning an additional language, such as English, are usually therefore caused by insufficient exposure to that additional language. More frequently, adults, including education staff, may have unrealistic expectations of a bilingual child. It is not possible for children learning two or more languages to progress at exactly the same rate as a child learning just one. This should not, however, be described as "language delay." Comparing bilingual children to monolingual children is one of the most common errors made by professionals. This is the reason that children who speak a home language should not be assessed using normative data that is based on monolingual English-speaking children. Not only is the total amount of language exposure for the additional language not comparable between monolingual and bilingual speakers, but the cultural barriers in the assessment materials are likely to disadvantage the bilingual child. This perspective only takes development in the additional language as important. Such an approach is inherently racist and ignores the value of the home language.

## Can children only have problems learning the home language, but not the additional language?

If a child appears to have stronger skills in their additional language compared to their home language this may be for several different reasons.

- The child does not really have difficulties with their home language but is reluctant to speak it in an assessment environment where they perceive that their home language is not appropriate or welcome.
- The child values the additional language more because of the high status of that language. As a result, the child speaks more additional language and begins to abandon their home language. This commences a pattern of language attrition, caused by a significant reduction or complete cessation of the use of the home language. This may even occur where parents do not speak the additional language. Language attrition may resemble language disorder.
- The child is perceived as bilingual due to their ethnicity or cultural group identity. However, they have been raised as a monolingual child only speaking the majority language, such as English.

## Key components of assessment of bilingual children

- Pre-referral
- The referral form and conversations
- The planning session – See "Working alongside interpreters"
- The initial assessment appointment
  - Parent interview
  - Language exposure and attitude questionnaire
  - Assessment of speech and language domains
- The debrief session – See "Working alongside interpreters"
- Onward referral and liaison with the multidisciplinary team – See the report template in the "Resources" chapter
- Clinical supervision – See "Barriers to working with bilingual children and how to overcome them"

## Pre-referral

Referring agents may include the child's parent(s)/carer, care-setting staff such as nursery workers, educational staff including teachers, and healthcare workers such as Health Visitors and GPs. In short, anyone who comes into contact with the child and family may refer the child to speech and language therapy services.

Regular referring agents should receive training on typical bilingualism and when to refer bilingual children for assessment of any possible speech, language, or communication needs (SLCN). In this way, the referrals are likely to be more accurate and ensure timely, early intervention.

Referrers should understand that:

- Concern about the language of education alone is not a sufficient basis to refer. The child should only be referred if they are unable to communicate their needs in both their home language(s) and the language of education. Additional language learning takes many years and will not develop at the same rate as monolingual children who have only been exposed to the language of education.
- If there are concerns about the child's abilities across both/all their languages, then referral should be made urgently. Many professionals adopt the "wait and see" approach, leading to much later referrals for bilingual children, especially for Speech Sound Disorder.

- Bilingualism will not have caused the speech, language, or communication needs. Parents need reassurance that their child would have experienced these difficulties regardless of the language background. This is important, as attitudes to the home language can influence the maintenance or loss of home-language skills.
- Many families will have had no experience of speech and language therapy services and may need an explanation of what the role is and what to expect.

## The referral form and conversations

In addition to the usual demographic information gathered for a referral to speech and language therapy services, it is important to ensure that the following is included on the referral form.

- The most frequently encountered languages in the catchment area
- The names of low-status as well as high-status varieties of languages spoken
- The need for an interpreter to be present at any appointments. It is extremely important to note that many professionals consider conversational English to be sufficient. This is not the case, and informed consent cannot be said to have been gained if a parent or guardian does not have excellent additional language skills. It is also important to consider that any carer in the household may wish to be present and will require an interpreter to be present.
- Availability on the telephone, or better still via video call. This will allow you to check that the interpreter's language skills match those of the family as reported on the referral form.
- All those involved in the care of the child or young person, including extended family members and the languages that they use with the child. It is common in many households for grandparents, older adult siblings, and others to take responsibility for childcare at different points in the day or week.

## Speech and language therapy referral form

| Child or young person's full name: | | | |
|---|---|---|---|
| Preferred first name: | | | |
| Date of birth: | | | |
| Date of referral: | | | |
| Sex assigned at birth: | Female | Male | Other: |
| Gender role: | Girl | Boy | Other: |
| Siblings' names, birth order and ages/date of birth: | | | |

*(Continued)*

(Continued)

| NHS number or Reference number: | | |
|---|---|---|
| Parent 1 name and role: | | |
| Parent 2 name and role: | | |
| Main carer: | | |
| Other carers:<br>*Include languages spoken with the child:* | | |
| Home language(s):<br><br>Tick ALL languages the child HEARS or SPEAKS<br><br>*Languages listed are commonly encountered in the UK. This is not an exhaustive list.*<br><br>*Please adapt to your catchment/ case load.* | Pakistani-heritage languages:<br>❑ Mirpuri<br>❑ Punjabi<br>❑ Urdu | Asian & African-heritage languages:<br>❑ Arabic<br>❑ Turkish<br>❑ Persian/Farsi<br>❑ Somali<br>❑ Tagalog/Filipino |
| | Bangladeshi-heritage languages:<br>❑ Sylheti<br>❑ Standard Bangla<br><br>Indian-heritage languages:<br>❑ Guajarati<br>❑ Tamil<br><br>Chinese-heritage languages:<br>❑ Putonghua<br>❑ Cantonese | European-heritage languages:<br>❑ English<br>❑ French<br>❑ German<br>❑ Italian<br>❑ Lithuanian<br>❑ Polish<br>❑ Portuguese<br>❑ Romanian<br>❑ Spanish<br>❑ Other: |
| Is an interpreter helpful for the assessment of the child, informed consent, and/or discussion with the parent(s)/ carer? | Yes | No |
| Heritage/Ethnicity: | | |
| Referrer's name: | | |
| Referrer's role: | | |
| Other professionals involved: | | |
| Has the child been referred previously? | No | Yes<br>Please provide details: |
| Current setting: | | |
| Medical diagnosis: | | |
| Reason(s) for referral: | | |
| Are there concerns about the child's ability to speak their home language(s)? | | |
| Are there concerns about the child's ability to speak the mainstream language/language of education? | | |
| What has been done so far to support the child? | | |

## Child or young person's name

It is important to note that not all cultures have the concept of a family or surname. Although many families begin to adopt the western style, many cultures give everyone a unique name. For example, naming convention for Pakistani-heritage children is often to use the father's first name as the child's last name, although this is not always the case.

Similarly, the child's first listed name may not be the name the child is referred to. Pakistani-heritage children may have a first listed name that is religious in nature, provided in honour of, for example, the prophet Mohammed (PBU). A child listed as *Mohammed Mustafa Waqas* is therefore likely to be called "Mustafa" by his family (and he will tell you he is called *Mustafa*), and his father is likely to be called *Waqas* (as his "first" or calling name). Note, that *Mohammed* is written first out of respect, but that the individual would never be called this name in any situation, except when formally writing or listed his name on official documentation. This [religious name] + [personal name] + [optional family or tribal/village name] may occur in any order (FBIIC, 2006).

Some last names are gender specific. For example, *Bibi, Begum* and *Khatoon* are feminine markers (Rahman, 2013, p. 257). It would be a mistake, therefore, to refer to Mrs Bibi's husband as Mr Bibi – "Mr Female-Person"!

There are also many variants to this convention, depending on the heritage and/or country of origin and family and cultural traditions. This is given as an example to illustrate that there are different naming conventions across cultures.

We have often encountered professionals calling children "Mohammed" (or worse, the colloquial "Mo") and being puzzled that the child doesn't respond. Some boys and men *do* use this name and take pride in it (Khaleeli, 2014), but it cannot be assumed that this is the personal name.

There are therefore no fixed rules to predicting the use of a person's name. **The best way to ensure you use the correct "first" or personal name is simply to ask the person or parent(s) and not to assume.**

## Date of birth

This may seem to be very straight forward. However, individuals may have been born in countries that did not have government infrastructure available to register births due to conflict or disaster (Sieff, 2013). Many immigrants are allocated the 1st January as their de facto birth date as the actual date is unknown (Business Insider, 2017). Some children and young people may not even know the exact year of their birth.

## Language(s)

On this form, the most frequently spoken languages in England and Wales (after English) are listed (ONS, 2013). In clinical practice, one would list the most frequently spoken languages in your catchment area. Data is available from local government sources and school language censuses. The service may also audit their referrals for the past 24 months and note which languages they encounter most frequently.

"Language" is not a simple term. Every language has a high-status form. This is often referred to as the "standard form" and is associated with power, politics, and privilege. In the UK, it is not accidental that "Standard English" is associated with the southeast, where Parliament, the BBC, and wealth are located in the capital city, London. People often place negative connotations on other regional dialects or accents, labelling them as imperfect, incorrect, or hard to understand. These associations lead to people who speak a less prestigious version of a language often incorrectly reporting that they speak the high-status variant. In addition, families from places with less well-known languages or language variants may assume that a white monolingual professional will not have heard of their language, and so agree that they speak the proffered well-known variant.

Stow (2006) found that only 45% of children referred to speech and language therapy services had their language correctly recorded. The other 55% often had a generic label such as the country of origin or heritage, such as "Pakistani" or "Chinese."

For these reasons, it is important to have a selection of the most frequently encountered languages and offer carers and parents a choice. That is (to a Pakistani-heritage family), "Do you speak Mirpuri, Punjabi, or Urdu?" rather than "Which language do you speak at home?" The latter is likely to elicit "Urdu," especially if asked by a white monolingual therapist, whereas citing the actual language will signal to the family that their language is valued and the difference from the standard language form is recognised.

"Dialect" and "accent" are not well defined (see the previous chapter for definitions of these terms).

## Parent 1 (and parent 2)

It should not be assumed that children or young people will have a mother and father. This is a cis-heteronormative idea that all caregivers are heterosexual and the same sex they were assigned at birth. Single parents, foster carers, individuals who adopt, same-sex couples, and transgender people are all carers, and clinicians will build a better relationship if they are open to these types of family structure, rather than just assuming roles. Many opposite-sex couples may include a new partner who is not the child's genetic parent.

## Parental or carer role

The use of "Parent 1" and "Parent 2" is not meant in any way to negate or eliminate the parent or carer's role. Rather, it reminds us to avoid making immediate assumptions based on gender and gender stereotyping. The name and role of each parent or carer should be recorded and used from that point onwards by the clinician in the case notes, reports, and other documentation. Many people, including both opposite-sex and same-sex relationships, may use home-language terms for the roles of "mother," "mama," "father," and "papa," for example, "Ami" and "Abba" (mother and father in Mirpuri). Other variants may also be valued and used by the family.

It is good practice to ask the name and relationship to the child/young person of **everyone** attending the appointment. Family friends, extended family, or other professionals may attend appointments. Each person's full name and relationship should be recorded in the case notes.

## Main carer

From a language exposure/input perspective, it is also useful to know who the main caregiver is, especially for children who are not attending a childcare or educational setting. Grandparents and older siblings may provide a very different language input than the parents. For example, it is very easy to assume when meeting two eloquent English-speaking parents that the child will mainly hear English. However, if the Mirpuri speaking grandmother is the main carer due to both parents working, then the child will likely speak Mirpuri as their main home language. Please see the *Language exposure questionnaire*.

## Other carers

Many extended families share childcare responsibilities, whether bilingual or not. Significant time spent with a carer who speaks a particular language should be considered.

Extended-family terminology may include labels which provide information on the family structure, where English labels may not. For example, in Mirpuri, the father's mother is "dadi" and the mother's mother is "nani." A list of Pakistani-heritage language (Mirpuri, Punjabi, and Urdu) family roles are listed at the end of the chapter as an illustration.

## Home language(s)

It is best practice to offer a choice of languages based on the most commonly encountered language spoken in the geographical area. These languages may be identified from neighbourhood statistics. Many families who speak less well-known languages or variants may report the better known and high-status variant. For example, Sylheti speakers may report that they speak Bangla, and Mirpuri speakers may report that they speak Urdu. This should be carefully explored. The interpreter will be able to identify if the language reported on the referral form is indeed the language being spoken by the family. There may well be codeswitching and attempts to use languages together to include all speakers.

> "The funny thing is, I can understand when my Mum and Grandad speak to me in Mirpuri, but when their Mirpuri friends come to visit, I don't understand a word! (That's when I realised that) my Mum and Grandparents speak to us in Mirpuri, they (codeswitch) words into Punjabi, so I can understand what they are saying. They just speak only Mirpuri with their Mirpuri friends, so I can't understand those conversations"
>
> *Bilingual Punjabi – English speaker discussing her*
> *family language usage.*

## The parent/carer interview (case history)

The interviewing of parent(s)/carer(s) of children to build a picture of the child's acquisition of speech and language to date is an important component of the assessment process. The is often referred to as the "case history." I avoid this terminology as it is derived from the medical model and, if used with parent(s)/carers, may be poorly understood.

As well as being culturally sensitive and inquisitive, SLTs may need to reassure parent(s)/carer(s) that home language is the best language to use during this process. Many individuals may feel that they can "get by" in English and want to demonstrate their competence in the language. Such speakers may feel patronised by the involvement of a professional interpreter. However, this ignores some key factors:

- Families who use home language will provide more detailed information in their home language, as they are not translating/filtering into English.

- The child, if present, should perceive the clinical space as a home-language environment. This will encourage home-language usage during any subsequent assessment tasks.

- The interpreter may have a more nuanced understanding of the child's strengths and needs when this is articulated by the family in their home language. The interpreter will also know if there are issues in translating low-frequency or technical terms, such as "stammering/stuttering" or "articulation."

- One parent/carer may be more confident in English than their partner. The use of English may therefore exclude one of the parents.

- Examples of the child's utterances, sounds, and so forth are likely to be in home language. It is harder to codeswitch and think of these examples, than when discussing the child's speech and language in the home language.

## Involving a professional interpreter

A professional interpreter should be involved unless the parent(s)/carer(s) both have a native level of English language. If the parent(s)/carer(s) object, the above points should be explained, and the fact that the interpreter is there to assist the child or young person and SLT, not the parent(s)/carer(s).

Further explanation that home-language assessment and therapy are the best course of action may also be helpful here.

## Eating and drinking

Food and drink are perhaps one of the main differences between cultures. Food is emblematic of certain countries and communities. In the UK, it is food that has been the leveller, with chicken tikka masala, a merging of the British love of gravy and curry, named the nation's favourite dish (Cook, 2001). Many other dishes from around the world, including pizza (Italian), chow mein (China), and hamburgers (Germany via the US), are widely popular. Despite this, few people have a detailed insight into the eating habits of other communities. It is important to be aware of what a typical family might eat and drink, and typical dining arrangements (not all children sit in a highchair nor join in at mealtimes with adults) and how this might impact on advice, especially for weaning and when dysphagia is suspected.

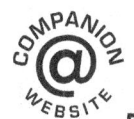
Adult informants from the community are ideally placed for this role. Professional interpreters will often have a great deal to offer in terms of insight into the culture they are a part of.

## Language exposure and attitude questionnaire

*It is recommended that you replace **"your child"** with the child's preferred name.*

*This questionnaire is a series of prompts for a conversation between the speech and language therapist and the parent(s)/carer of a child or young person, typically alongside an interpreter. Consider that many parent(s)/carers will find reading and/or writing in English very challenging or impossible, so always work alongside an interpreter presenting the questionnaire verbally in the home language unless you are certain that the parent(s)/carer has a very high literacy level in English.*

| 1. | Which language(s) is/are heard and used at home? <br> a) Please list all languages spoken or heard in your home: | | | |
|---|---|---|---|---|
| | b) Between parent(s)/carers when talking together? | | | |
| | Between siblings (brothers, sisters)? | | | |
| | Name of brother or sister | Age (Years) | Language(s) spoken | Language(s) spoken with [your child] |
| | | | | |
| | | | | |
| | | | | |
| | | | | |
| | By grandparents and other relatives such as aunties, uncles, and cousins with [your child]? | | | |
| | Other people who regularly speak with [your child]? <br> *Consider video and telephone calls* | | | |
| | Care/Educational setting (Nursery, School, College etc.) | | | |
| 2. | Which of these languages are used to speak directly to [your child]? <br> • Consider: <br> ○ which person speaks which language to the child? <br> ○ for what purposes? Think of mealtimes, play and education activities | | | |

| 3. | Do you have a language policy?<br>*Do you have **rules** about which languages may be spoken at home versus outside the home, which everyone knows and follows?*<br><br>❏ Home language at home and with extended family and friends/Mainstream language outside or in work and educational settings<br>❏ Both/all languages spoken in all settings<br>❏ No policy/never discussed this |
|---|---|
| 4. | Which language(s) do you wish [your child] to be able to use when they are 18 or older?<br><br>❏ Home language(s) ❏ Mainstream language (such as English)<br>❏ Other<br>❏ Don't know<br><br>*Discuss that, unless home language is used daily, it is likely to be lost through language attrition.* |
| 5. | Are you worried that speaking home language(s) will slow down their education?<br>❏ YES<br>❏ NO<br>❏ Don't know<br><br>*Provide information and reassurance that this is NOT the case* |
| 6. | Are you worried that using home language(s) with [your child] has caused or contributed to their speech/Language Difficulties?<br>❏ YES<br>❏ NO<br>❏ Don't know<br><br>*Provide information and reassurance that this is NOT the case* |
| 7. | What are [your child]'s three longest spoken sentences? This might include examples where [your child] uses both/all languages within the same spoken sentence (codeswitching).<br>*Provides information on current ability to use expressive language*<br><br>1)<br>2)<br>3) |
| 8. | How does your child ask for food, drink, or snacks? |
| 9. | Does [your child] speak in the same way as other children his age?<br><br>❏ YES – Speaks well in both/all languages<br>❏ NO – Home language is not as good as other children their age<br>❏ NO – Mainstream/Language of Education (such as English) is their best language<br>❏ NO – Speaks two or more languages but overall cannot get their message over in the same way as other bilingual children their age |

*(Continued)*

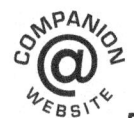

(Continued)

| | |
|---|---|
| 10. | Does [your child] use words from two or more languages in their spoken sentences (utterances)?<br><br>❏ YES – They use words from both/all their languages<br>❏ Not applicable – They only use home language<br>❏ Not applicable – They only use the mainstream language/language of education (such as English)<br>❏ Not applicable – they are not using *complete* spoken sentences yet and miss out important parts of the spoken sentence (such as the person or action, or omit words or word endings)<br><br>*Explain that codeswitching is a sign of typical language development in bilingual children and not a sign that the child is confused by hearing two or more languages* |
| 11. | How long has [your child] attended school?<br><br>Did they attend school in another country and/or in another language previously? |
| 12. | Does [your child] attend a Saturday/Weekend/Evening school where they speak a home language, or another language (other than the mainstream language) with other children?<br>❏ YES<br>❏ NO |
| 13. | Does [your child] learn a language/learn to recite a language for religious purposes?<br>❏ YES<br>❏ NO<br><br>Is this language used for conversations or for reciting prayer/religious texts?<br>❏ Used as a language for conversations<br>❏ For religious purposes<br><br>Do they have difficulties remembering the religious texts?<br><br>❏ YES – they cannot remember it all<br>❏ YES – they stammer/stutter/get stuck<br>❏ NO – they can remember all the prayers and texts when given enough time to practice<br><br>*Consider arranging a visit to the religious setting to discuss the child's needs and explaining that speech, language, and communication needs are not associated with the child or young person being disrespectful.* |
| 14. | Does [your child] play with other children from the neighbourhood?<br>Which language(s) do they speak together?<br><br>❏ YES – The children speak home language(s) together only<br>❏ YES – The children speak mainstream language together only<br>❏ YES – The children speak both home language(s) and the mainstream language<br>❏ NO – My child only plays alone or with siblings<br>❏ DON'T KNOW |

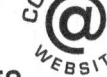

| | |
|---|---|
| 15. | Does [your child] watch television/downloaded programmes and films/movies, and/or play video games?<br><br>❑ NO<br>❑ YES<br><br>In which language(s) are these programmes/films/movies/video games?<br><br>How long does [your child] spend on these activities per week? |
| 16. | Does [your child] ever refuse to speak home language(s)?<br>*If so, is this because of the place, the person they are speaking to, or the activity they are undertaking? Consider the pragmatics of the person and setting. For example, nursery and school may be considered a strictly mainstream language environment.*<br><br>❑ NO - They are happy to speak home language(s) most or all of the time<br>❑ YES - They won't speak home language(s) outside of the home<br>❑ YES - They won't speak home language at school/educational settings<br>❑ YES - They won't speak home language(s) with some people: |
| 17. | Does [your child] answer in the mainstream language (such as English) when you speak to them in home language?<br><br>❑ NO - They always reply in home language(s)<br>❑ YES<br><br>If so, how do you deal with that situation?<br><br>*Provide advice on re-modelling spoken utterances that the child uses in the mainstream language into home language to help the child or young person understand that home language should be spoken in the home environment.* |

## Assessment domains

Which areas to assess will be guided by the concerns highlighted by referring agents and parent(s)/carers. However, routine screening is recommended for all domains to ensure that the child has sufficient skills across all speech and language areas.

A screen is a quick task which acts to confirm that there are no apparent difficulties in that domain. Should the child have significant difficulties, then a more in-depth full assessment may be undertaken. A diagnosis should not be based on screening level assessments alone.

For bilingual and multilingual children, the SLT should undertake assessment of both/all languages that the child is exposed to.

**Table 3.1** Factors supporting home-language development or driving language attrition and loss

| Factors supporting home-language(s) maintenance | Factors driving home-language attrition and loss |
|---|---|
| Home-language usage policy: Everyone is expected to speak home language | Home language is used by parent(s)/carer and child replies in mainstream language |
| Home language(s) is/are spoken by all adults, even if they are fluent in mainstream language | Home language is only spoken by one parent/carer |
| Siblings use home language with the child | Older siblings use mainstream language only |
| Films/movies/music and games, books and/or stories and other fun activities are provided in home language(s) | Fun activities are in the mainstream language (films/movies/music/games) and discipline and chores are discussed in home language |
| Regular contact with relatives who speak the home language(s) such as extended family, video and telephone calls, visits to relatives in the heritage country/countries | No contact with heritage culture |
| Family members are keen to maintain their cultural heritage and value their home language | Family is keen to integrate into the mainstream community and believe that differences may lead to poor educational outcomes; discrimination and/or bullying |
| Intervention and home practice is carried out in home language(s) | Speech Sound Disorder or (Developmental) Language Disorder is incorrectly associated with home-language usage and so the family switch to mainstream language only |

Tick the boxes to ensure that you have assessed each domain across both/all languages.

- For multilingual children, add additional columns for each language heard/spoken.
- For additional investigations, add rows. For example, fluency.
- Informal, culturally adapted assessment materials are superior to translated published assessments.

## Decision making

The SLT has several key decisions to make when first information gathering and assessing the bilingual child. These include:

1. Which language should assessment be carried out in?
2. Which language should intervention/treatment be carried out in?
3. Is the child developing speech and language skills like other bilingual children of this age, or is there a speech and/or language disorder present?
   *This is the "differentiating disorder from diversity" question*

**Table 3.2** Assessment summary

| Domain | Home language/ Mother tongue | Mainstream language (such as English) |
|---|---|---|
| Language: Verbal comprehension<br>*Following spoken instructions*<br>*Parent/carer reporting* | | |
| Language: Expression<br>*Use of spoken language*<br>*Language sample* | | |
| Language: Listening vocabulary<br>*Selecting words from a choice of items* | | |
| Language: Naming vocabulary<br>*Confrontational naming* | | |
| Speech: Articulation<br>*Stimulability of single phones*<br>*Check phone inventory for that language* | | |
| Speech: Phonology<br>*Word naming and connected speech sample* | | |
| Phonological awareness skills<br>• *Clapping out syllables*<br>• *Discrimination (same/different)*<br>• *Identification (matching or sorting sounds to pictures/articulograms)*<br>• *Onset-rime*<br>• *Phoneme isolation*<br>• *Segmentation*<br>• *Alliteration* | | |
| Other domains<br>*Please state:* | | |

4.  Is the child likely to continue using home language, or lose the home language through attrition?

To answer these questions, we must consider the outcomes for the child and family.

## Language dominance

Many clinicians believe that if a child is already dominant in the mainstream language (such as English), that it is permissible to carry out assessment and intervention in the mainstream language. This is often based on false logic.

*Apparently dominant in the mainstream language due to pragmatics associated with the setting and/or person assessing*

If the SLT assesses the child or young person in an educational setting, then the child is likely to associate that setting with the mainstream language (typically English). Speaking home language(s) may seem wrong or unusual, especially as a clearly monolingual professional is present.

Young children may not be aware that their languages are different on a conscious level, especially where their language community frequently uses codeswitching. I have assessed children where they have used English words and phrases, and when asked, denied that they were English words and phrases. Bilingual children may view their languages in the same way that a monolingual speaker consider synonyms.

In order to encourage the child to use home-language skills,

- Assess at home, either in person or via telehealth
- Always work alongside a professional interpreter
- Plan the session with the interpreter so that from greeting to undertaking tasks, only home language is used.
- Undertake "warm-up" activities such as a game, picture storybook (that is culturally appropriate), or conversation about favourite foods, for example. This will signal that the situation is a home-language one.
- Carry out several informal visits where you engage in play activities in home language prior to undertaking the assessment.
- Flag up any mainstream language responses and have these re-phrased in the home language by the interpreter. For example:
  - Child: "I like milk."
  - Interpreter: "Meh dood passander."

*Dominant in English and experiencing language attrition at home*

Children sense that English and other mainstream languages are high status. This is unsurprising. Mainstream languages such as English feature in nursery rhymes, games, television, films/movies, video games, books, websites, and other internet-enabled entertainment, and they are the language of children's teachers. This leads to the odd phenomenon where children speak English to their parent(s)/carer, even if the parent doesn't understand English. We have observed this especially when children have just started in a care or educational setting.

This disconnect between the parent(s) home language use and mainstream acquisition by the child can eventually lead to the child being unable to speak the home language, and the parent unable to speak to their child in the mainstream language. This isolation from primary carers is highly damaging to children and young people and should be avoided at all costs.

Many politicians have stated that to avoid this, parents should learn the mainstream language. The need to learn the mainstream language is not disputed but learning the mainstream language should not involve the loss of home language and the associated loss of cultural identity that follows. There are often barriers to learning the mainstream language, especially for women.

## Family language policy

The home language policy (whether this a conscious decision, or a result of changing circumstances) should be discussed. A family language policy is how the family decide to balance the use of languages, considering social, emotional, practical, and cultural aspects.

The most commonly employed is the one-person one-language approach (OPOL) (Danjo, 2018). This approach has been criticised as it is based on the idea that the child may be confused by hearing two languages used together, and that parents fail to implement the policy, even when they are committed to it, as bilingual people are often unaware of their code-switching behaviours (Goodz, 1989).

The family language policy best suited to avoid language attrition is to use home language(s) within the home, and the mainstream language at school and outside the home. There may be some exceptions, such as only using home language(s) with a person who cannot speak the mainstream language or using the mainstream language to discuss homework. The family should explore the best options for them, focusing on the outcome that the child should be able to speak the language they would have spoken if a speech, language, or communication need had not intervened. Aspects to consider are:

- The **person's current language abilities**
- The **overall amount of language exposure** to ensure opportunities for acquisition
- The **activity** being undertaken
- The **location** and the child's perception of which language(s) can/should be spoken there
- The **people** present. Visitors for example may trigger a change in language. Siblings who are older may peer the mainstream language and need reminding to use their home language skills.

**Table 3.3** List of terms to denote relationships in Pakistani-heritage languages: Mirpuri, Punjabi, and Urdu

**Terms listed in the order:**
**i) Mirpuri ii) Punjabi iii) Urdu. If only one listed then same lexical item for all three languages**

*Immediate family*

| # | Nearest English equivalent | i) Mirpuri  ii) Punjabi  iii) Urdu |
|---|---|---|
| 1. | Father | aba |
| 2. | Mother | ʌmi |
| 3. | Brother | pəɾa / pəɾa OR paɾʼi / bʰʌhai |
| 4. | Sister | pɛn / pɛn / bʰen |
| 5. | Son | pʌt̪ʃ / pʌt̪ʃ / bet̪a |
| 6. | Daughter | t̪i / t̪i / bet̪i |
| 7. | **Older brother** *Also used for unrelated people who are older than you* | papa / bʰʌhai d͡ʒan *literally "brother-dear"* / bʰʌhai d͡ʒan *literally "brother-dear"* |
| 8. | **Older sister** *Also used for unrelated people who are older than your* | bad͡ʒi OR d̪ed̪i / bad͡ʒi OR apã / bad͡ʒi OR apã |
| 9. | **Brother-in-law** | *See older brother if older than you* |
| 10. | **Sister-in-law** | pabi / pabi / bʰabi |
| 11. | **Nephew** (Brother's son) | bət̪ɛɾie / bət̪id͡ʒa / bət̪id͡ʒa |
| 12. | **Nephew** (Sister's son) | bʌnija / bʰand͡ʒa / bʰand͡ʒa |
| 13. | **Niece** (Brother's daughter) | bʌt̪ɛɾi / bʌt̪id͡ʒi / bʌt̪id͡ʒi |
| 14. | **Niece** (Sister's daughter) | bʌne / bʰand͡ʒi / bʰand͡ʒi |

*Extended family – Aunts, Uncles, and Cousins*

| # | | | i) Mirpuri  ii) Punjabi  iii) Urdu |
|---|---|---|---|
| 15. | **Paternal Uncle** *Father's brother* | a. Older than father | t̪aja / t̪aja |
| | | b. Younger than father | t̪aja |
| 17. | **Paternal Aunt** *Father's sister* | | puwa OR pupi / puwa OR pupi / pupi |

**Spouse**

| # | | | i) Mirpuri  ii) Punjabi  iii) Urdu |
|---|---|---|---|
| 16. | **Aunt** *Father's brother's wife* | a. Older than father | t̪aji / t̪aji |
| | | b. Younger than father | t͡ʃat͡ʃi |
| 18. | **Uncle** *Father's sister's husband* | | pupa OR t̪aja *if paternal aunt is older than father;* OR t͡ʃat͡ʃa *if paternal aunt is younger than father* / pupa / pupa |

| # | Relation | | | | # | Relation | |
|---|---|---|---|---|---|---|---|
| 19. | **Maternal Uncle** *Mother's brother* | mamu: OR maɳa | mamu: OR mama | mamu: | 20. | **Aunt** *Mother's brother's wife* | mami: OR maɳi: / mami: / mami: |
| 21. | **Maternal Aunt** *Mother's sister* | hala or ma'si → halu or maɳa | hala or ma'si → halu | hala → halu | 22. | **Uncle** (Mother's sister husband) | halu or maɳa / halu / halu |

|  |  | | | |
|---|---|---|---|---|
| 23. | **Cousin** | [Uncle] + plural + / [Aunt word] + | na (male); OR | + mʊrɑ (boy) — e.g., ʈɑjai na mʊrɑ *Father's older brother's son* |
| | | | ni (female) | + kʊri (girl) — e.g., puwa na mʊrɑ *Father's sister's son* |
| | | [Uncle] + plural + / [Aunt word] + | ɖa (male) | + mʊnɖa (boy) — e.g., mame ɖi kʊri *Mother's brother' daughter* |
| | | | ɖi (female) | + kʊri (girl) — e.g., hala ɖi kʊri *Mother's sister's daughter* |
| | | [Uncle or Aunt word] + | zaɖ | + [brother] or [sister] |

*Extended family – Grandparents*

| # | | | | Spouse | | |
|---|---|---|---|---|---|---|
| 24. | **Grandfather** *Father's father* | ɖ aɖ a | 25. | **Grandmother** (Father's mother) | ɖ aɖ i |
| 26. | **Grandfather** *Mother's father* | nana | 27. | **Grandmother** (Mother's mother) | nani |
| 28. | **Child** | bʌt͡ʃa (male) / bʌt͡ʃi (female) | 29. | **Children** | bʌt͡ʃae |
| 30. | **Elderly man** | baʋa d͡ʒi / baba d͡ʒi / baba d͡ʒi | 31. | **Elderly lady** | bei d͡ʒi |

## References

Business Insider. (2017). *Here's why a lot of immigrants have birthdays on January 1st. YouTube.* www.youtube.com/watch?v=L0t1SDtdBUQ

Cook, R. (2001, April 19). Robin Cook's chicken tikka masala speech. *The Guardian*, Thursday. www.theguardian.com/world/2001/apr/19/race.britishidentity

Danjo, C. (2018). Making sense of family language policy: Japanese-English bilingual children's creative and strategic translingual practices. *International Journal of Bilingual Education and Bilingualism*, 1–13. https://doi.org/10.1080/13670050.2018.1460302.

Financial and Banking Information Infrastructure Committee (FBIIC). (2006). *A guide to names and naming practices.* www.fbiic.gov/public/2008/nov/Naming_practice_guide_UK_2006.pdf.

Goodz, N. S. (1989). Parental language mixing in bilingual families. *Infant Mental Health Journal*, *10*, 25–44. https://doi.org/10.1002/1097-0355(198921)10:1%3C25::AID-IMHJ2280100104%3E3.0.CO;2-R.

Khaleeli, H., & Henley, J. (2014, December 1). Muhammad: The truth about Britain's most misunderstood name. *The Guardian*, Monday. www.theguardian.com/uk-news/2014/dec/01/muhammad-truth-about-britains-most-misunderstood-baby-name.

Office for National Statistics (ONS). (2013). *2011 census: Quick statistics for England and Wales, March 2011.* ONS. www.ons.gov.uk/peoplepopulationandcommunity/populationandmigration/populationestimates/bulletins/2011censusquickstatisticsforenglandandwales/2013-01-30.

Rahman, T. (2013). Personal names and the islamic identity in Pakistan. *Islamic Studies*, *52*(3/4), 239–296. www.jstor.org/stable/43997225

Royal College of Speech and Language Therapists (RCSLT). (2022). *Clincial guidance: Bilingual guidance.* https://www.rcslt.org/members/clinical-guidance/bilingualism/bilingualism-guidance/

Sieff, K. (2013, December 31). In Afghanistan, Jan. 1 is everyone's birthday. *The Washington Post.* www.washingtonpost.com/world/in-afghanistan-its-everyones-birthday/2013/12/31/81c18700-7224-11e3-bc6b-712d770c3715_story.html

Stow, C. (2006). *The identification of speech disorders in Pakistani heritage children.* University of Newcastle. http://theses.ncl.ac.uk/jspui/handle/10443/1588

# WORKING ALONGSIDE INTERPRETERS

DOI: 10.4324/9781003125563-4

# Working alongside interpreters

Most people still say "using an interpreter." This phraseology ignores the complex and challenging role of the interpreter. The interpreter is asked to do the impossible: Make one person's spoken utterances in one language sound like an analogous utterance in another language. Think about that for a moment. What's the Russian equivalent of "It was raining cats and dogs" or "Don't throw the baby out with the bathwater"? You may be unfamiliar with these eccentric British idioms yourself. Bulkes and Tanner (2016) created a database of 870 American English idioms, and so they seem to be a relatively frequent feature of English.

However, as we shall see, it is not just esoteric sayings such as these that are a challenge to the interpreter. Even a single word can involve multiple decisions, with a very different outcome than a monolingual English speaker might expect. Interpreters are therefore making unconscious and conscious decisions based on many factors, including their role, who they are translating for, and how much knowledge they have about the speakers and the purpose of the question. Interpreters are a valuable member of the multi-disciplinary team and central to working with bilingual children and their families.

## Advantages of working alongside an interpreter

Working alongside an interpreter greatly improves the quality of communication, understanding and bridging of cultural barriers and leads to better professional relationships. The superior clinical outcomes delivered illustrate the false economy of working exclusively in the majority language (Acar & Blasco, 2018).

## Locating a home language interpreter

If the interpreter service is not able to provide a local interpreter, consider requesting an interpreter elsewhere who can assist via telehealth. This is a far preferable option than accepting that no one is available and working only in English (or the language of education).

## Matching an interpreter

Some authors have recommended matching the therapists' and interpreters' gender to the parent's gender. This is not always possible, especially if both parents are of a different gender. In my experience, questions such as those surrounding childbirth and breastfeeding are not embarrassing for female parents when the reason these questions are being asked is carefully explained via an interpreter in home language, rather than an abrupt question being asked. The parent interview (case history) should be a conversation conducted with sensitivity. As a gay cis-male SLT, I have never had a mother refuse to see me due to my gender. As a respected professional, it is the presence of an interpreter and sensitivity to culture and home language which are important. In common with any other appointment with a health professional, the option to bring along a chaperone is good practice and should be made clear at the pre-assessment video/voice call.

It is good practice to check with the parent(s) if they have a preference for the gender of the interpreter (NHS England, 2018). For some parents, especially those who are refugees and may have experienced violence or sexual assault, a contact with a home language speaker of a particular gender may be triggering and traumatic. This should be documented in the case notes and signalled on the front of the case notes so that any future contacts involve checking that the interpreter booked for appointments is of the preferred gender.

## Three-way telephone interpreting and telehealth

Services are available where an interpreter translates between the SLT and the service user over the telephone. These types of service may be helpful for:

- checking the home language(s) are correct
- providing urgent information and advice
- providing information on speech and language therapy (what it is, as some families may not have encountered the profession before, or it may be unavailable in their home country)
- providing information on where and when to attend (location of the clinic, for example)
- reassuring the family that an interpreter will be present at the planned appointment.

Due to the complexity of communication and assessment, and the practical difficulties of assessing young children, it is unlikely that a whole episode of care could be delivered over the telephone.

Since the COVID-19 pandemic, many more families and professionals have become familiar with telehealth, where professionals and families communicate via a video call. This has obvious advantages over the telephone, and many services delivered successful assessment and therapy when no other in-person options were available.

Telehealth continues to offer advantages where no local interpreter is available. Assessment and therapy via telehealth in home language will be preferable to an English-only approach.

It is worth noting that some families will face barriers accessing telehealth including financial barriers such as the costs of Wi-Fi or calls where Wi-Fi is not available or affordable. Some families may have no suitable hardware such as a smartphone, tablet, or laptop/desktop computer. Similarly, some parents and carers may not have the technical skills to use software and equipment. Although these problems are less frequent, it should be considered that one or more of these barriers may prevent a family from accessing care via telehealth.

## Difference between an interpreter and a translator

An interpreter works with people via spoken language. A translator works with written language. SLTs typically work only with interpreters. Working with translators may be required for producing materials such as reports, or for AAC. However, when considering written materials such as appointment letters, information leaflets, care plans and therapy programmes, SLTs should consider videos and/or audio recordings of the interpreter explaining these materials as the default way of delivery.

## Identifying the correct language and dialect

Communities are often grouped together by heritage. For example, Bangladeshi-heritage people or Pakistani-heritage people. This may even lead to referring agents using generic terms such as "Chinese," "Pakistani," or "Bangladeshi" as languages, obscuring the rich diversity of languages spoken within those communities. More importantly for the work of the SLT, where exact translation may be crucial, the wrong language may be identified. Stow (2006) found that only 45% of Pakistani-heritage children had their language correctly identified on the referral form to speech and language therapy services.

"Dialect," "accent," and "slang" have very different meanings compared to those used within English. A person with a southern English accent in England will be able to identify that they are speaking to a speaker with a northern English accent, but will not have any difficulty understanding the speaker. Differences tend to be in some vowels and a small number of lexical items, which may be easily guessed from the context.

In contrast, a "dialect" in a language may be actually describing a completely different language that is not mutually intelligible to speakers of other "dialects." This was noted in a survey of people who accessed interpreter services: "People were also concerned about language proficiency in terms of their own mother tongue. Bangladeshi and Gujerati people, for example, felt that service providers often were unaware of the range of different Asian languages and dialects within each language" (Alexander et al., 2004, p. 19).

> "[The Pakistani heritage languages Mirpuri, Punjabi and Urdu] . . . they are completely different languages. People really can't understand each other [from these different language communities]. It's not just a little change, it's quite a big gap."
>
> *Zahida Warriach, Senior Bilingual Speech and Language Therapy Assistant*

SLTs should therefore research the languages and any "dialects" spoken by families in their area. These variants should be offered so that parents and carers can select the correct language(s) spoken by the family. Lists of languages may be found by consulting local and national census data and languages spoken in local school.

## Bilingual speech and language therapy assistants and bilingual co-workers

People with bilingual skills may not have previously considered the role of SLT, or speech and language therapy assistant. In the UK, speech and language therapy is the least diverse of the allied health professions, with less than 5% male and 3.5% Asian, 1.3% Black, and 1.9% "Other ethnicity" (Moore et al., 2020). This compares to national figures of 8% Asian, 3.5% Black, and 1.9% other ethnicity (ONS, 2021). Although it is important to acknowledge that ethnicity does not equate with bilingualism, the figures demonstrate that the profession does not reflect the population we serve.

Attracting bilingual speakers to these roles requires active recruitment from these communities. Simply using the term "Bilingual" on a job advert may be enough to prompt interest (rather than just advertising for a SLT or Assistant post).

> "Because suddenly people that wouldn't dream of applying for a speech therapy assistant post will start applying because they perceive themselves to have bilingual skills and therefore they'll go for it, whereas they might discount their bilingual skills and say I haven't got the skills that you need to be a speech therapy assistant."
>
> *Dr Carol Stow, Consultant Speech and Language Therapist*

> "(I had) No idea what I was going for. It said 'Bilingual Co-worker' and so I applied."
>
> *Zahida Warriach, Senior Bilingual Speech*
> *and Language Therapy Assistant*

As mentioned previously, one assistant cannot hope to speak all the languages spoken in the local area, so why employ a speaker of only one of those languages?

> "Just having a bilingual assistant in the department who speaks any language is an advantage because they ... change the mindset of that department. Because they suddenly start to open your eyes to the fact that there isn't just one way of doing things. That not everybody eats the same food, eats the same food at the same time, using the same cutlery, that they don't relate to different generations in the same way, that their acceptance of particular toys or their perception of children (may be different to those of monolingual English speakers)."
>
> *Dr Carol Stow, Consultant Speech and Language Therapist*

This exploration of cultural knowledge and challenging monolingual cultural assumptions is explored in more depth elsewhere in this book.

## Different types of literacy: language learning for religious purposes

Some communities may learn to decode the written text of a language in order to access religious texts. An example of this is Muslim non-Arabic speakers who engage in religious study of the holy Qur'an. Muslims believe that the Qur'an was revealed to the prophet Mohammad (PBUH) in Arabic and is literally the word of God. Therefore, to change the language would be to change the word of God. The Qur'an is therefore read in the original Arabic language.

As Muslims who speak Pakistani-heritage languages such as Mirpuri, Punjabi, or Urdu cannot understand Arabic, learning the Qur'an is a matter of memorising passages by rote and/or decoding Arabic text semi-phonetically.

> "[As young children] ... we're just basically rote learning with no idea what we're saying ... As you get older, into your teenagers or adults, what people tend to do is they buy the Quran with the [Urdu] translations underneath the Arabic text [in order to understand the meaning]."
>
> *Zahida Warriach, Senior Bilingual Speech and Language Therapy Assistant*

It is a mistake, therefore, to claim that such people "speak Arabic." In the same way that a Christian might recite Latin, there is no functional everyday understanding and use of Arabic. The language is reserved for religious purposes.

Other religious communities have similar language learning expectations, although the language used in religious ceremonies and functions may range from being limited to such functions right through to being a functional everyday community language.

Children with dysfluency (stammer or stutter), or who have difficulty with literacy or short-term memory (such as those with Speech Sound Disorder or Developmental Language Disorder) may have significant difficulties with the task of rote learning. The SLT has a role to inform and educate religious leaders and teachers who hold religious lessons about speech and language disorders. This will allow reasonable adjustments to be made for such children and young people and dispel the false impression that they may be being disrespectful or unruly.

## Myth: bilingual SLTs don't need an interpreter

Bilingual or multilingual SLTs are able to work with the communities with which they share a language. In some countries, this may be sufficient to reach the whole of the local population. However, in the UK and most other multicultural societies, the sheer number of different languages spoken means that the bilingual SLT will not be able to provide a service without the assistance of an interpreter.

## Who should work as an interpreter?

Children and young people under the age of 18 years of age should never work as/act as an interpreter. Such children are likely to miss out on their own education if brought to appointments to act as an interpreter. While they may have sufficient language skills to translate in everyday activities, they are unlikely to have the skills to understand or be able to translate the complex technical language encountered in a speech therapy session (consider for example the difference in meaning between "speech" and "language"). In addition, these young people may suffer trauma being the first person to receive complex information about lifelong diagnoses and having to relate that information to their parents.

Similarly, adults who are not qualified or paid as professional interpreters should not be asked to leave their roles in order to act as an interpreter. For example, a bilingual person working in a community clinic may be asked to act as an interpreter causing them additional work and stress. Non-professional interpreters are also likely to be unaware of the need for confidentiality.

It is also possible that child protection issues are raised during an appointment or contacts with a bilingual child or young person.

## Who is the interpreter for?

Working with interpreters may be prevented by one or more of three main barriers:

- The cost of the interpreter is challenged by a manager or team lead
- One or more parent/carer feels patronised as they can speak both their home language and the language of the appointment (typically English)
- The family can speak English to a level where they can "get by"

The interpreter's role is to ensure that all family members including the child or young person, and the professionals are included as fully as possible. Even if one or more parent/carer feels that their English is at a high level, a session carried out exclusively in English is not desirable for the following reasons:

- **Using English only will mark the clinical setting as a monolingual English-speaking environment.** The child will perceive it as pragmatically inappropriate to speak their home language and so be reluctant to speak the home language when required to do so during an assessment. This often leads to a false assumption that the child is now "dominant in English" because they "choose" to speak only English. The reality is that the child is conforming to the pragmatic constraints set by the situation. This is an example of unconscious bias towards the language of education.
- Parent(s) and carers are more likely to provide accurate information about the child's abilities in their home language when discussing this in the home language. The parent(s)/carer can provide examples of the child's speech and language in home language, including first words and utterances, where appropriate. It is much more natural to consider the child's home language utterances when discussing this topic in her language. The alternative would be to codeswitch, and although codeswitching is frequent in bilingual communities the dominance of the English language makes this more challenging.

"They (a South Asian person) can come in quite tense. And then suddenly the body language changes, and they become relaxed . . . I think it's really building that communication for them, to really let you know how they feel about their child's speech and language needs and what their worries are and their concerns."

*Zahida Warriach, Senior Bilingual Speech and*

*Language Therapy Assistant*

*Cost of working with an interpreter*

In the UK, the Equality Act (2010), the NHS constitution, NHS clinical guidelines, and RCSLT clinical guidelines all highlight that access to an interpreter is an essential component to providing care to bilingual individuals and their families. SLTs who do not comply with these guidelines risk working outside of their professional boundaries, and if challenged may discover they are therefore uninsured should they be subject to disciplinary action for acts of omission.

For those SLTs working in private practice, it is important to emphasise that the provision of an interpreter should not be optional when working with such families and clients. The cost of an interpreter should be included in the overall care package. Private practitioners may feel under pressure to remove the need for an interpreter in order to keep costs down for the family. This is a false economy as the poor outcomes for the client and family are not worth the saving. In addition, the clinical outcome will almost certainly result in the child or young person losing their home language via language attrition. This often inadvertent outcome may not have been discussed with the family and may cause severe distress and isolation from the family and community.

Providing a service only in the mainstream language or language of education (typically English or Welsh) is an example of structural racism and should be strongly challenged, as this is neither evidence based nor equitable.

## "Getting by" and informed consent

One or more parent/carer may feel patronised by being offered an interpreter. It should be made clear that it is not the intention to question someone's ability to speak English. Rather, the interpreter is there in order to assess the child's speech and language abilities in her language, and to offer support to all family members present at the appointment.

Many families who spend the majority of the time speaking home language, but do use English for basic needs such as informal chats, shopping, and other every day activities, may feel that they have a fair to good level of additional language skill. However, this may be insufficient to understand complex terminology, life changing diagnoses, and negotiating care packages and educational placements for children and young people with additional needs.

The SLT and other professionals need to ensure that they have a very high level of confidence that information and choices they are discussing with parent(s)/carers are completely understood. Without this level of confidence, we cannot claim to have gained informed consent from parents/carers.

For this reason, it is important to work alongside interpreters for assessment, intervention, and meetings with parents/carers. This includes multidisciplinary meetings and those carried out in educational and care settings. Should an SLT or other professional attend a meeting where an interpreter is not present, they should ensure that the parent is able to provide informed consent. If there is any doubt, or if a parent has previously worked alongside an interpreter, then the meeting should be rearranged until an interpreter has been booked for the meeting.

## Child protection and interpreters

Bilingual children and young people may not be able to report abuse due to a language barrier combined with a speech, language, or communication difficulty. In addition, bilingual children may be unfamiliar with the role of professionals and the range of services available to assist them.

Interpreters should be adults over the age of 18, have references, and/or be employed by an organisation that has carried out checks on their professionalism and language skills. Interpreters should receive mandatory training on child protection, understand confidentiality, and have been cleared for work with children and young people (such as the enhanced Disclosure and Disbarring Service (DBS) in the UK) (Cambridgeshire & Peterborough Safeguarding Partnership Board, 2022). When this guidance is not followed, many barriers arise which may lead to a failure of the child protection procedure (See Chand, 2005).

Disclosure of anything which puts a client/patient in potential harm, physically, emotionally, sexually, or financially, should be reported to the appropriate services. Please refer to Child Protection and Vulnerable Adults policies and procedures, and any other relevant safeguarding procedures.

Should a bilingual patient/client make a disclosure in home language, **the interpreter or bilingual co-worker must be involved in reporting the disclosure** in their capacity as a professional. Interpreters or other suitably qualified bilingual co-workers **should be involved in all stages of safeguarding procedures,** to ensure that the client/patient's disclosure is understood and that they are kept informed at all times, as appropriate.

In rare circumstances, one parent/carer may object to an interpreter being involved as part of controlling behaviour, isolating the abused adult. The presence of an interpreter may allow the abused parent/carer to ask for help. Adult safeguarding procedures should be consulted if an adult seeks help during an appointment. It is therefore important that professional interpreters are aware of such policies and have training on both adult and child protection.

## A timetable for SLTs working alongside interpreters

Most SLTs currently work in an ad-hoc way, assuming that interpreters will know how to work with families from their community. Although this may be true, many interpreters will only have a hazy idea of the role of the SLT and what they aim to achieve within any particular session. Add to this the complexity of cultural and linguistic differences, and failure to plan may lead to errors, confusion, and poor outcomes.

## Double the time essential for equitable outcomes

The RCSLT states that in order to achieve the same clinical outcomes, SLTs working with bilingual families should have double the time compared to working with a family with whom they share a language (Royal College of Speech and Language Therapists [RCSLT], 2021). This approach is consistent with other caring professions, where the process of working alongside an interpreter and addressing cultural barriers took double the time (Eklöf et al., 2015). Guidelines on the commissioning of services also highlights the need for "typically double that of a regular appointment" (NHS England, 2018, p. 6).To fail to provide this would be another example of institutional racism.

## Translation of written materials

Many SLTs try to make their service accessible by translating information leaflets, signage, and providing care plans and activities in the family's home language. This is costly and may be ineffective for many communities.

Providing written information in home language is appropriate for families who come from highly literate societies, where access to education is universal. For other families, there may be several barriers to accessing written information.

**Table 4.1** Time allocation when working with bilingual children and young people and their families

| Step | Description | People involved | Suggested time allocation[1] | Main tasks |
|---|---|---|---|---|
| 1. | Making **initial contact** with the family via three-way telephone interpreting service or telehealth appointment alongside an interpreter. | SLT and interpreter | 20-30 minutes | • Check the language on the referral is correct.<br>• Offer a choice of languages (dialects)<br>• Explain what will happen at the appointment.<br>• Explain what speech and language therapy is.<br>• Check the family know where/how to attend. |
| 2. | **Planning** the **initial appointment**, including parent/carer interview and direct assessment of the child's speech and language skills in home language. | SLT and interpreter | 60 minutes | • Transcribe greetings in home language(s) for the SLT to say to the family, signalling a home language environment and welcoming the family<br>• Identify non-standardised assessment materials that are culturally appropriate<br>• Transliterate questions, prompts, and targets for any expressive language assessment<br>• Discuss the purposes of assessment and translation style:<br>  ○ Free translation style for parent/carer interview<br>  ○ Close/detailed translation style for language assessment<br>• Demonstrate transliteration for the interpreter and check their competence in transliteration. |
| 3. | **The initial appointment** Home language assessment | SLT and interpreter, child/young person, and parent(s)/carers | 1-4 appointments 60-90 minutes each | • Parent/carer interview in home language<br>• Transliteration of expressive language sample in home language<br>• Speech sound assessment in home language<br>• Assessment of any other relevant domains of speech and language<br>• Provide initial advice through home language using a verbal medium |
| 4. | **The initial appointment** Mainstream language assessment | SLT and interpreter, child/young person, and parent(s)/carers | 1-4 appointments 60-90 minutes each | • Assessment of expressive language in mainstream/additional language<br>• Assessment of speech sounds in mainstream/additional language<br>• Assessment of any other relevant domains of speech and language |

| Step | Description | People involved | Suggested time allocation[1] | Main tasks |
|---|---|---|---|---|
| | | | | • **NB.** The interpreter is still present to support the child/ young person to understand instructions and to support the parent/carer who may not have sufficient English to engage effectively. |
| 5. | **Observation in the home** (Where appropriate) Home language | SLT and interpreter, child/young person, and parent(s)/ carers. Possibly sibling(s) and home language- speaking friends/peers. | 60 minutes plus travel time | • Observe free play, routine, and interactions in home language.<br>• Observe interactions with sibling(s) and peers in home language.<br>• Observe other aspects of speech, language, and communication, as well as eating and drinking as appropriate. |
| 6. | **Observation in school/ educational setting** (Where appropriate) Mainstream language (Typically English/ Welsh) | SLT and teacher, teaching assistant, and/ or Special Educational Needs Coordinator. Child/young person. Parent(s)/ carers may wish to meet you at the end of the session alongside the interpreter. | 60 minutes plus travel time Additional time for liaison with staff. | • Observation of interactions with education staff (adults) and peers in additional language<br>• Observation of any strategies the child/young person uses such as imitating others' actions, or asking for help from a home language speaker |
| 7. | **Diagnosis, report discussion and arranging intervention and/or onward referrals** | SLT and translator. SLT and interpreter. | 60-90 minutes | • Information on the diagnosis and supportive organisations should be provided in a verbal as well as written format. A video of the interpreter working alongside the SLT made by parent(s)/carer may be appropriate here.<br>• Report in written English/ Welsh provided so parent(s)/ carers can share with other professionals.<br>• Verbal format report provided by an interpreter (recorded by parent(s)/carer for later reference and sharing with the extended family)<br>• Professional translated report on request (especially for speakers with high literacy levels).<br>• Informed consent for onward referrals gained in home language |

*(Continued)*

**Table 4.1** (Continued)

| Step | Description | People involved | Suggested time allocation[1] | Main tasks |
|------|-------------|-----------------|------------------------------|------------|
| 8. | **Planning home language intervention** | SLT and interpreter. Consultation with parent(s) to include their ideas and address any concerns. | 60-240 minutes | • Looking up any available data on speech/language development in home language(s)<br>• Liaison with a specialist adviser<br>• Devising aims and therapy tasks based on available information about home language(s)<br>• Identifying culturally appropriate therapy materials<br>• Writing transliterated questions and likely responses into informal recording forms<br>• Making home language, home practice materials |
| 9. | **Home language intervention** | SLT and interpreter Parent(s)/carer | 60-90-minute sessions. Typically, episodes of care will take double the monolingual allocation to achieve the targets. Episodes of care under 8 weeks are likely to be ineffective | • Carry out the programme with the interpreter proving a translation of instructions and comments. Parent(s)/carer video this session for later reference and sharing with the extended family, should they wish to.<br>• Consider observing the parent(s)/carer delivering the home practice activities in home language so that you can provide feedback on treatment fidelity. |
| 10. | **Mainstream language intervention and advice** | SLT and education staff Parent(s)/carer | 60-90 minutes plus travel time | • Provide information on strategies to deliver a language-rich environment in the classroom<br>• Explain the maintenance/restoring of home language<br>• Explain the difference between typical additional language learning and a core speech, language, or communication disorder<br>• Discuss the possibility of delivering home language intervention via a bilingual teaching assistant |
| 11. | **Outcome appointment** | SLT and interpreter | 1-2 appointments of 60-90 minutes | • Gather the impressions and reports of the child's progress or failure to progress. Request specific examples of words, phrases and utterances used.<br>• Adaptation into home language of a parent reported outcome measure such as the FOCUS (Thomas-Stonell et al., 2013)<br>• Explanation of any outcomes and revised action plan, or discharge as appropriate. |

| Step | Description | People involved | Suggested time allocation[1] | Main tasks |
|------|-------------|-----------------|------------------------------|------------|
| 12. | **Discharge** | SLT and interpreter | 60–90 minutes | • Explanation of the decision, such as the child is now using language at similar levels to their bilingual peers.<br>• Explanation and copies of any discharge report or letters and who will receive them.<br>• Request for written translations if the parent(s)/ carer are literate in their home language.<br>• Verbal translation of the discharge report delivered by the interpreter and videoed by parents.<br>• Written information and verbal translation of how to request re-access/rereferral to the service. |

[1] For an experienced Specialist SLT. More junior staff, students and those new to working with bilingual families may take as much as double this time allocation. More complex cases, or those with more team members involved may take more sessions.

Pre-planning session

However, there is an assumption that written materials can be translated into all other languages, and that this is an effective way to meet the needs of non-English speakers. This viewpoint has been challenged for many decades, with the recognition that many people cannot read English or their home language (Tuffnell et al., 1994), and that verbal translation is a much more effective way of providing information.

This is made even more urgent, when considering that many phrases and technical terms may have no analogue in home language or may be poorly translated and culturally insensitive (Shaw & Ahmed, 2004). "Technical terms" may be as simple as there being no easy way to differentiate terms such as "word" and "sound," as well as names for conditions such as "stammering/stuttering." Examples, when not from the targeted community, may cause confusion. Arora et al. (2012) found that "some foods, drinks and dietary habits appropriate to Western culture may be unheard of, or contrary to traditional Chinese health beliefs" (537).

*Pre-literate languages (language with no written form)*

Some communities either have no written form for their language (preliterate) or have poor access to education and so cannot read their script. This is often true for girls (who later become mothers), who may have had limited or no education due to the exclusion of girls from education.

Service providers often default to the high-status written text, even when people with related languages cannot understand those high-status languages. For example, providing Urdu written information to Mirpuri speakers is unlikely to lead to complaints, as Urdu is seen as a formal and educated language, used by the powerful and elite, but these speakers would still need assistance via verbal interpretation to understand such information.

*Low levels of literacy associated with deprivation*

Literacy levels are low for all populations (including monolingual) in areas of deprivation. It is estimated that more than a quarter of working aged adults (16-65 years) have low literacy or numeracy skills or both (Kuczera et al., 2016).

In summary, information is best provided in-person alongside an interpreter in order to clarify any problems regarding technical terms and cultural misunderstandings. Rather than pay for written translations of appointment letters, information leaflets and care plans, SLTs should record the interpreter and make the video/audio available to the family. For more general information, demonstrating therapy techniques, or providing information, these videos could be published on websites and linked with QR codes for ease of access. It is far less embarrassing for a parent/carer to request help with translating an English text than their home language text.

## Providing information, intervention, and reports via video format

Accessibility should therefore be the default position.

The NHS provides guidance on translation. This includes ensuring that access to information around health care is provided free to service users. Services can also request that information is provided in a verbal format in the language of their choice. This is known as "sight translation" (NHS England, 2018).

Information technology and the widespread availability of high-quality audio video equipment in the form of tablets, mobile telephones and other devices mean that it has never been easier to share information in formats other than the written word.

It is sensible to default to verbal means of communication. SLTs should check that they have identified the correct home language. Interactions alongside an interpreter will confirm that the adults providing care for the bilingual child are able to understand and use their home languages to a high degree of sophistication.

Many families now have access to tablets and smart phones, and are able to use these devices to access the internet. This allows SLTs and other professionals to provide rapid links to resources using QR codes so that parents and carers do not have to type in long links. There are numerous free websites where any URL may be converted to a QR code. The QR code can then be added to a leaflet, linking a video of an interpreter providing a verbal translation in home language so that both the parents and the wider family may access a verbal presentation of that printed material/written material.

Part of the planning when working with a family should be time to record such resources. For example, before giving a diagnosis of language disorder, the SLT should record the information leaflet provided to monolingual English speakers being translated by a professional interpreter into home language.

Clear advantages are apparent for enabling people within the home to deliver any intervention activities in home language. For example, aunties, uncles, older adult siblings, grandparents, and other members of the extended family may wish to work with the child in the home language. Providing a video demonstrating activities in home language alongside an explanation of the reasoning behind these activities increases the pool of adults who are able to act as support in delivering treatment and as being role models in using home language with the child.

## The use of computerised translation apps and services

Even with human translators, examples of cultural insensitivity and inaccuracy of technical terms is commonly encountered (Acar & Blasco, 2018; Shaw & Ahmed, 2004). The risk of this is even higher with artificial intelligence.

Many services send data for translation outside of the European Union for processing. It is not always possible to see how the app or service is processing data. There are also risks of data being intercepted by third parties when transmitted across the internet via an unencrypted route. In the UK, this would likely breach the Data Protection Act (2018).

**Figure 4.1** Example of a QR code linking to a leaflet on bilingualism

The service may select the wrong language. Written-language varieties are often the high-status version, as they are linked to education, politics, and power. Those families speaking other languages such as Sylheti or Mirpuri will likely not be able to read high-status written languages such as Standard Bangla and Urdu. So, carrying out the translation may be pointless.

Finally, the rise of real-time computerised interpretation on smart devices has become a reality. This method may miss subtle clues that the parent, carer, or child is uncomfortable, nervous, or anxious. A real-life interpreter would pick up these non-verbal and verbal signals, and difficult issues such as child protection may arise. These clues would be lost if using a computerised service. Again, the highly confidential data may be transmitted unencrypted anywhere across the internet, posing a risk to confidentiality.

For these reasons, the Royal College of Speech and Language Therapists does not recommend the use of these apps and services.

## Seating position when working with an interpreter

The interpreter is the voice of the SLT. The situation should never be a relay between the therapist, the interpreter, and the home-language speaker(s). Rather, the SLT should make eye contact with their conversational partner (the client/carer/child) and speak directly to them. In this way the conversation is directly with the home-language speaker(s) and not a conversation with the interpreter.

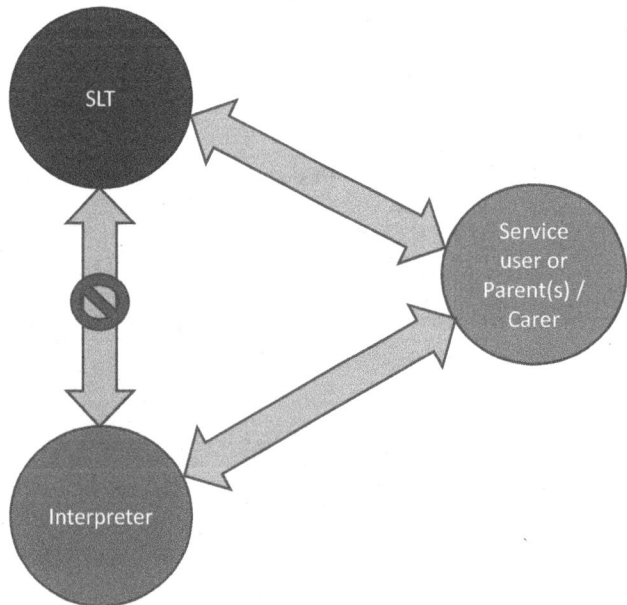

**Figure 4.2** Seating position when working with an interpreter

The room and seating should be set up so that all three people can be comfortably seated within an imaginary triangle. The SLT should speak, pause, and wait for the interpreter to deliver the interpreted spoken utterance. Hearing the reply from the home-language speaker, the therapist should wait for the interpreted spoken utterance to be delivered in English (or their language), while continuing to look at the client/carer.

Some practitioners prefer to have the interpreter sitting next to them so that they can maintain eye contact with the parent or service user.

## Tips for working alongside an interpreter

- **Book twice the time when working with a bilingual family** as you would usually for a monolingual family with whom you share a language (typically English).
- **Plan the session.** Always have time to discuss the expected tasks during the session, the cultural appropriacy of any toys, pictures, and other materials, and any questions the interpreter may have.
- **Speak at your normal speaking volume.** Do not raise your voice or over articulate. The interpreter should ensure that the home-language speakers(s) understand anything you choose to say.

**Table 4.2** Incorrect examples of working with an interpreter

| | |
|---|---|
| *Therapist to interpreter:* | *Can you tell them that my name is Sean and I'm the speech and language therapist?* |
| Interpreter to mother: | *Verbal translation provided* |
| Therapist to interpreter: | Now tell them your name and what your role is. |
| Interpreter to mother: | *Verbal translation provided* |
| | Can you tell them that the teacher has asked me to see their child because they're worried about their talking? |
| Interpreter to mother: | *Verbal translation provided* |
| Therapist to interpreter: | How does she feel about his talking? |
| Interpreter to mother: | *Verbal translation provided* |

**Table 4.3** Correct examples of working with an interpreter

| | |
|---|---|
| *Therapist to mother:* | *Hello, my name is Sean and I'm the speech and language therapist.* |
| Interpreter to mother: | *Verbally translates the above* |
| Therapist to mother: | This is Saba, the interpreter. |
| Interpreter to mother: | *Verbally translates the above* |
| | (Your child)'s teacher has asked me to see (your child) because they're worried about their talking. |
| Interpreter to mother: | *Verbally translates the above* |
| Therapist to mother: | How do you feel about their talking? |
| Interpreter to mother: | *Verbally translates the above* |

- **Speak at a relaxed pace.** Keep a warm and calm demeanour, and show that you are interested in the family and happy to help them. Many bilingual families are faced with impatience when trying to communicate. Make the appointment as stress-free as possible.

- **Look directly at the person you are conversing with, the service user or the parent(s)/ carer.**
  Do not look at the interpreter unless you are saying something directly to them for their attention.

- **Introduce yourself and everyone present.**
  Say what your professional role is and what this involves. Many families will be unfamiliar with professional roles, or incorrectly expect a medical intervention.

- **Ask each home language speaker to introduce themselves and their relationship to the child or young person.**
  Is the person accompanying the child the mother, auntie, or other extended family member?

- **Discuss confidentiality.**
  The family may be concerned that their personal and private information will be discussed with others in the community. This can be concerning, especially if the family are refugees and fear professionals are unsympathetic government agents, or if there is a small community and they know the interpreter. You may have to arrange another interpreter if the interpreter is known to the family for this reason. Inform the family that the interpreter is bound by professional confidentiality and will face sanctions if they talk about the appointment to others.

- **Do not promise absolute confidentiality.**
  Explain that you will keep all conversations and information confidential, except where child or adult safeguarding means you may have to ask other professionals to help.

- **Use short, simple sentences, and provide examples of any technical words, concepts, or phrases.**
  Avoid asking a series of two or more questions. Technical terms may include what speech and language therapy is or words such as "sound," "word," "stammering/stuttering," "phonology," "disorder," and so forth.

- **Include everyone in the conversation.**
  There may be a family dynamic where some members speak the mainstream language well and feel that an interpreter is not required. You should explain that the interpreter is there so that everyone is included and that you can work with the child or young person in home language(s). If that person then tries to monopolise the conversation by answering your questions before they have been translated acknowledge

that response but still wait for the translation to be completed and then listen to any response that this elicits in home language from other family members present.

- **Make sure that everything said in the room is translated.**

  This includes phrases such as "I'm just going to the photocopier" or similar. A home language speaker will be much more relaxed if they can follow the whole conversation and translating everything means that they are not excluded.

- **Keep control of the conversation.**

  This is a session for you to find out about the family, or carry out assessments or therapy tasks. You should expect a pattern of:
  - The SLT speaks in English (or mainstream language)
  - The interpreter provides the home language equivalent
  - The child, young person or parent/carer speaks
    The interpreter provides an English translation

  Do not allow free conversation to develop between family members and the interpreter or family members. This will result in very large sections of translation, and details will be lost.

- **Ensure that the interpreter is not asked inappropriate questions.**

  There is a risk that the interpreter will be asked personal or off-topic questions, such as how they got the job, where they live etc. This is often the case with female interpreters, where working may be less acceptable in some cultures.

- **Ensure that parent(s)/carers are signposted to other services.**

  It is the role of the SLT to ensure that everything is translated and that you are able to signpost to other services, should parents/carers ask the interpreter, such as family planning, GP clinics, advice on passports, residency, and other concerns.

- **Monitor speech directed to children and young people.**

  Children and young people may have parents offering rewards or punishment in home language if they do or do not answer questions or complete tasks. Some cultures may interpret failure to comply as defiance on the part of the child or young person and wish to ensure that their child is responding politely. This may be to miss a comprehension problem, lack of confidence in responding to adults, or even a block for a person with a stammer (dysfluency). Ensure everything is translated so that you can help parent(s)/carer to understand how to offer appropriate rewards or respond in an encouraging way.

- **Use a free translation style for interviews (case history).**

  This style of translation means that the interpreter is free to paraphrase and provide the most accurate answers to your questions in spoken sentences that are well formed in both languages.

- **Use a close or detailed translation style for expressive language assessment.**
  This style of translation involves morpheme-by-morpheme translation that is technical and preserves the clinical data.
- **Do not write down a translation of the child or young person's utterances. Rather, write down a transliteration of the utterance using English letters (English orthography).**
  This can be carried out by the SLT or interpreter. See the *Translation Protocol* (Pert & Stow, 2003).
- **Book the same interpreter across the whole episode of care, if possible.** The interpreter will get to know the family and develop trust and rapport. The SLT will not need to keep updating a new person or explain the role of the team and assessment or therapy aims.
- **Debrief the interpreter.**
  This allows discussion after the family have left. Any transliterated language data can be translated and discussed. Issues or concerns can be discussed and clarified. **Plan the next session** before the interpreter leaves for their next appointment.
- **Thank the interpreter.**
  They may be being paid for their work, but this is unlikely to be highly paid work and many people work in healthcare interpreting out of social responsibility and a wish to assist members of their community. This work can be demanding, requiring good concentration skills, as well as emotionally taxing.

## References

Acar, S., & Blasco, P. M. (2018). Guidelines for collaborating with interpreters in early intervention/ early childhood special education. *Young Exceptional Children, 21*, 170–184. https://doi.org/10. 1177/1096250616674516.

Alexander, C., Edwards, R., Temple, B., Kanani, U., Zhuang, L., Miah, M., & Sam, A. (2004). *Access to services with interpreters: User views.* Retrieved February 13, 2022, from www.jrf.org.uk/sites/ default/files/jrf/migrated/files/1859352294.pdf

Arora, A., Liu, M. N. M., Chan, R., & Schwarz, E. (2012). 'English leaflets are not meant for me': A qualitative approach to explore oral health literacy in Chinese mothers in Southwestern Sydney, Australia. *Community Dentistry and Oral Epidemiology, 40*, 532–541. https://doi.org/10.1111/ j.1600-0528.2012.00699.x

Bulkes, N. Z., & Tanner, D. (2016). "Going to town": Large-scale norming and statistical analysis of 870 American English idioms. *Behavior Research Methods, 49*, 772–783. https://doi.org/10.3758/ s13428-016-0747-8

Cambridgeshire & Peterborough Safeguarding Partnership Board. (2022). *Working with interpreters and other with special communication skills.* Retrieved February 13, 2022, from www.safe guardingcambspeterborough.org.uk/children-board/professionals/procedures/working-with-interpreters-and-others-with-special-communication-skills

Chand, A. (2005). Do you speak English? Language barriers in child protection social work with minority ethnic families. *The British Journal of Social Work, 35*, 807–821. https://doi.org/10.1093/bjsw/ bch205

Data Protection Act. (2018). *Data protection act 2018.* GOV.UK. Retrieved February 16, 2022, from www.gov.uk/government/collections/data-protection-act-2018

Eklöf, N., Hupli, M., & Leino-Kilpi, H. (2015). Nurses' perceptions of working with immigrant patients and interpreters in Finland. *Public Health Nursing (Boston, Mass.), 32*, 143–150. https://doi.org/10.1111/phn.12120

Kuczera, M., Field, S., & Windisch, H. C. (2016). *Building skills for all: A review of England. Policy insights from the survey of adult skills.* OECD. www.oecd.org/education/skills-beyond-school/building-skills-for-all-review-of-england.pdf.

Moore, I., Bitchell, L., & Lord, R. (2020). *The health & care professions council equality, diversity and inclusion data 2020 report.* Health & Care Professions Council. Retrieved February 13, 2022, from www.hcpc-uk.org/resources/reports/2020/edi-data-2020-report

NHS England/Primary Care Commissioning. (2018). *Guidance for commissioners: Interpreting and translation services in primary care.* NHS England. www.england.nhs.uk/publication/guidance-for-commissioners-interpreting-and-translation-services-in-primary-care

Office for National Statistics (ONS). (2021). *Population estimates by ethnic group and religion, England and Wales: 2019.* Retrieved February 13, 2022, from www.ons.gov.uk/peoplepopulationandcommunity/populationandmigration/populationestimates/articles/populationestimatesbyethnicgroupandreligionenglandandwales/2019

Pert, S., & Stow, C. (2003, September 5–7). *A translation protocol for speech and language therapists.* 5th CPLOL Conference. www.research.manchester.ac.uk/portal/en/publications/a-traceable-translation-protocol-for-speech-and-language-therapy-teams-working-with-bilingual-clients (89991c4f-9f91-4da5-90db-c9fa8e1ef5cf).html.

Royal College of Speech and Language Therapists (RCSLT). (2021). *Clinical guidelines: Bilingualism guidance.* Retrieved January 16, 2022, from www.rcslt.org/members/clinical-guidance/bilingualism

Shaw, A., & Ahmed, M. (2004). Translating genetics leaflets into languages other than English: Lessons from an assessment of Urdu materials. *Journal of Genetic Counseling, 13*, 321–342. https://doi.org/10.1023/B:JOGC.0000035525.68249.52

Stow, C. (2006). *The identification of speech disorders in Pakistani heritage children.* Doctor of Philosophy, University of Newcastle. http://theses.ncl.ac.uk/jspui/handle/10443/1588

Thomas-Stonell, N., Oddson, B., Robertson, B., & Rosenbaum, P. (2013). Validation of the focus on the outcomes of communication under six outcome measure. *Developmental Medicine and Child Neurology, 55*, 546–552. https://doi.org/10.1111/dmcn.12123.

Tuffnell, D. J., Nuttall, K., Raistrick, J., & Jackson, T. L. (1994). Use of translated written material to communicate with non-English speaking patients. *BMJ, 309*, 992–992. https://doi.org/10.1136/bmj.309.6960.992.

# TRANSLATION PROTOCOL

DOI: 10.4324/9781003125563-5

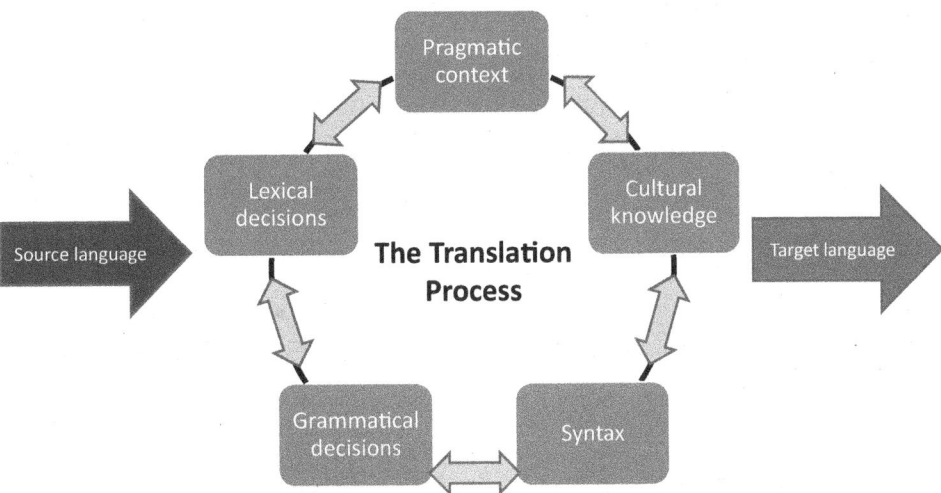

**Figure 5.1** The translation process model

## Translation styles

There are different styles of translation:

- A more natural, fluid style is appropriate while interviewing (or "taking a case history," in medical phraseology). This is a "free translation" style.
- When discussing proposed activities and outcomes with a child's family a more precise style is needed for language samples. These will form the basis for decisions regarding the child's diagnosis and the therapy which flows from that diagnosis.

This chapter presents a suggested translation protocol which allows accurate recording of a child's language sample and therefore supports accurate diagnosis and therapy.

## Taking a language sample

A language sample should be representative of the child or young person's ability, allowing the speech and language therapist to evaluate expressive language skills on several levels, including:

- Syntax: the arrangement of phrases
- Grammar: the acceptability of the utterance to a native listener (Crystal, 1988), often expressed as rules, but more accurately is a judgement of whether the utterance expresses the speaker's intentions.

- Morphology: the shape of word elements that encode ideas such as gender, number, and time (tense)
- For bilingual speakers: Codeswitching: the acceptable inclusion of content words from other languages whilst maintaining the grammar of the utterance frame.

Informal measures such as Mean Length of Utterance (MLU) may also be calculated. Unlike mainstream languages, especially English, the language under examination may be underdescribed in the literature. Many languages, especially community languages such as Sylheti and Mirpuri, have only recently been described in detail. This also does not include language contact situations in which two languages are in constant close proximity, such as Mirpuri and English in the UK, where changes may take place making both the Mirpuri and English less like the standard or home-language versions spoken in monolingual contexts.

A language sample might be gathered through an informal play session, in response to illustrations or photographs, or during another activity familiar to speech and language therapists. For bilingual children, the clinician also needs to consider:

- **Will the child or young person recognise the activity or objects in the picture?**
  Examples include Pakistani-heritage children in England not being familiar with knives and forks, as eating with the hands and roti (traditional flatbread) is more frequent.
- **Will the child be familiar with the assessment situation?**
  Children may not be used to adults allowing the child to take a lead. Stow et al. (2012, p. 26) found, "In many families, children are not expected to initiate communication with adults, and when addressed by an adult, children are expected only to give a concise and prompt response, not always verbal. As a result, children may fail to respond because of these pragmatic differences, or offer a non-verbal response such as eye pointing."
- **Will the child understand that home language is required?**
  - Children may not realise that they speak two or more different languages. Adults in the community may frequently codeswitch, and this is seen as the norm.
  - The pragmatic situation may encourage children to use one of their languages most strongly associated with that setting. For example, English for school, and Mirpuri for home.

## The use of transliteration to record home language responses

Transliteration is where the alphabet of one language is used to write down what is said in another (Merriam Webster, 2022). The result will not be entirely consistent as different speakers will have slightly different ways of encoding a particular word. However, this slight disadvantage is overshadowed by the huge advantage of having accessible text that any colleague can read and then discuss with the family and interpreters.

For speech and language therapists, a written record of what a child or young person says in home language is vital. A translated version will often be inaccurate, or credit the child with elements that they have not actually employed. For example, in Mirpuri "kha-na" means literally "eat + present progressive + male gender of the person eating." This single-word utterance might be translated as "he is eating" by an interpreter keen to get the best possible meaning across. From a speech and language therapist's perspective, the child has used a pronoun, an auxiliary, and three words! The role of the interpreter, to facilitate smooth understanding, has compromised the data whilst attempting to be as helpful as possible. Without the source data, the speech and language therapist cannot hope to analyse even single-word utterances.

The second problem is that the speech and language therapist cannot read all the possible alphabets available. Tens or hundreds of languages might be spoken in the local geographical area. If the interpreter wrote in their own alphabet and script, this might be an accurate record of the utterances the child produced, but it is likely inaccessible to the speech and language therapist who doesn't speak or read that language. Some languages don't have a written form.

To overcome this, transliteration using the (English) Roman alphabet is recommended for language samples.

For phonetic and phonological transcription and analysis, this should be carried out using the International Phonetic Alphabet (IPA) (International Phonetic Association, 2015). This is, however, less challenging as these samples are usually single words and short phrases, whereas a language sample may be numerous multi-word utterances.

## A suggested protocol

The following protocol was designed by speech and language therapists working with languages other than English on a routine basis (Pert & Stow, 2002, 2003). The protocol is designed to allow the evaluation of the spoken utterance as discussed above.

## Source language

The source language is the language you hear the child or young person speaking. This will be home language for most assessments, for example, Mirpuri.

## Target language

The language into which the utterance is to be translated. This is the mainstream language, typically English.

## Prompts and strategies

"Forced alternatives," where the child is presented with a choice of response is a strategy frequently employed by SLTS. In a survey of 536 UK SLTs, forced alternatives were the second most frequently employed strategy after modelling (Roulstone et al., 2012).

Providing a model ("modelling") was the most frequently employed strategy.

**Table 5.1** Expressive language recording grid

| | |
|---|---|
| **Adult home language utterance:** <br> *Target sentence* | |
| **Translation:** <br> *morpheme-by-morpheme direct translation* | |
| **Target translation:** <br> *Best analogue in English/Mainstream language* | |
| **Child/Young person's utterance:** <br> *Transliterated verbatim in roman letters* | |
| **Morpheme-by-morpheme translation:** <br> *Best analogue in English/Mainstream language preserving home language word/phrase order* | |
| **Closest English translation:** <br> *Best analogue in English/Mainstream language using English/Mainstream language syntax and grammar* | |
| **Clinician's comments:** <br> *Differentiation between an acceptable synonym, different way of expressing the target utterance, and obvious errors and omissions which would not be acceptable to a home language-speaking adult* | |

**Key**

- (E) lexical item said in English/(MSL) lexical item said in mainstream language
- (H) Home language, where "H" is the home language label, For example, (M) for Mirpuri
- Item in brackets, e.g., (he) = item is not omitted from the home language utterance but there is no analogous item in English, and this is the nearest/best translation.
- Bespoke key items explaining the mapping of home language morphological elements onto English or the Mainstream language. Examples for Mirpuri translated to English are shown.
- F/alt = Forced alternative provided in home language, for example, "Is this a *girl* or *boy*?" This notation should differentiate spontaneous expressive language from that imitated after an adult model.

**Table 5.2** Examples of morphological mapping

*Mirpuri Source to English Target Language*

| | |
|---|---|
| + male ➔ (he) | Grammatical element of present progressive agreeing with the gender of the subject of the sentence. |
| + female ➔ (she) | Grammatical element of present progressive agreeing with the gender of the subject of the sentence. |
| + respect ➔ (they) | Respectful grammatical marker with literal translation of "they" is not translated literally but marked for function. |
| (the) or (a) | Articles which are included in the translation to provide a complete sentence and indicate that there is **no omission** in the source language, but that determiners and articles **do not exist** in the source language. |
| () | Any item which has meaning marked in the source but has no analogue in the target language. |

**Table 5.3** Example of Mirpuri expressive language samples translated into English

| Adult home-language utterance: | kʊɾi | t͡ʃal | maɾ-ni | pi |
|---|---|---|---|---|
| **Translation:** | girl | jump | do-(contact) – ing + female | is + female |
| **Target translation:** *Best analogue in English/ Mainstream language* | *(the) girl (she) is jumping* | | | |
| **Child/Young person's utterance:** | **"girl jump maɾ-<u>na</u> pi-ja"** | | | |
| **Morpheme-by-morpheme translation:** | (E) girl (E) jump do-ing + male is + male | | | |
| **Closest English translation:** | (the) girl (he) is jumping | | | |
| **Clinician's comments:** | **Syntax:** Frame and phrase order taken from Mirpuri, AGENT – PATIENT – ACTION (Surface form *Subject + Object + Verb*. Please see the chapter on *Language assessment and intervention in home language* for a full explanation of the term "Frame" and the thematic roles "Agent," "Patient," and "Action.") **Grammar:** "jump" is a noun + generic verb phrase in Mirpuri, "maɾ-," which denotes contact/hitting/striking (legs hit the ground) **Lexical:** the child has codeswitched the AGENT and ACTION into English but retained the syntax – Typical codeswitching. **Morphology:** The child has used the gender agreement to denote a male AGENT, instead of a female AGENT in error. Utterance not acceptable – agreement error | | | |

## Areas to be considered during the translation process

### Lexical Items (Semantics)

- What's the nearest referent, most commonly used?
- Codeswitching is typical, and words from different languages may be used as synonyms by the child or young person. Young children may be unaware which language a lexical item comes from when asked.

- Have words been borrowed from a language in close contact and replaced the home-language word?

  For example, in Mirpuri-English, /bɔlə/ (from "ball") has replaced the home-language word /geṉḍ /.

- Is the choice of word influenced by other items in the utterance?
- What are the other choices?

  For example, in Mirpuri, "ʌs-na" is "smile-ing + male," but also "laugh-ing + male." The semantic boundaries to signify happiness encompass both *smiling* and *laughing*.

- Is the word part of an idiom or phrase where the meaning is conveyed over a phrase?

  For example, "It's raining cats and dogs" (It's raining hard).

- Does the language have decorative, cultural, or playful elements which do not contribute to meaning but are aspects of pragmatics and culture?

  For example, rhyme, cultural references, or non-standard forms.

- Is there a key item which changes the meaning completely?

  For example, "She put up the picture"/"She put up **with** the picture"

- Is the word/phrase a religious or cultural formality?

  This may involve the use of a whole phrase used as a frozen unit akin to a word, such as "How do you do?" (Hello/Greeting).

  British Muslims would usually use the greeting "Asalaam alaikum," which is an Arabic phrase linked to their religious identity, even if they speak no Arabic in their everyday life outside of religious devotion (Jaspal & Coyle, 2010).

### Grammatical features (Morphology/Phrase level)

- Where are grammatical features indicated?
- At the beginning of words?
- At the end of words?
- As separate words? (Do native speakers perceive these as separate words?)
- Are there variations according to time (tense), gender (of the subject/object), and number?

### Context, Social Norms, or Acceptability

- Ellipsis and Context – also consider that the source language may also be able to indicate features in different ways

  e.g., "Coffee?"

  "What's the man doing?" – "eating a banana"

  (Mirpuri speakers would know if it were a male or female who is eating)

**The translation process is not linear – all these levels influence each other**

**Table 5.4** Example of errors in home language – gender agreement

| | | | |
|---|---|---|---|
| **Adult home-language utterance:** *Target sentence* | kʊɾi | betʰ-i | vi |
| **Translation:** *morpheme-by-morpheme direct translation* | girl | sit - ing + female | is + female |
| **Target translation:** *Best analogue in English/Mainstream language* | (the) girl (she) is sitting | | |
| **Child/Young person's utterance:** *Transliterated verbatim in roman letters* | "girl beth-a va" | | |
| **Morpheme-by-morpheme translation:** *Best analogue in English/Mainstream language preserving home language word/phrase order* | (E) girl sit-ing + male is + male | | |
| **Closest English translation:** *Best analogue in English/Mainstream language using English/Mainstream language syntax and grammar* | (the) girl (he) is sitting | | |
| **Clinician's comments:** *Differentiation between an acceptable synonym, different way of expressing the target utterance, and obvious errors and omissions which would not be acceptable to a home language-speaking adult* | • Phrase order correct for Mirpuri (Mirpuri frame)<br>• Normal codeswitch of AGENT to English "girl"<br>• Correct lexical verb<br>• Incorrect use of male gender agreement on lexical verb, and incorrect gender agreement on the auxiliary | | |

Note that in the above example, it is not possible to express the error of gender agreement satisfactorily in English. The nearest we can get is "(he)," since the gender agreement is not a lexical item (pronoun) in its own right. The home language-speaking adult would perceive this as an incorrect or ill-formed utterance.

## Differences between languages and codeswitching

Codeswitching within a spoken utterance (intrasentential codeswitching) is common in many bilingual communities, especially where there is a long history of language contact with the mainstream language.

The surface form of a spoken utterance may be misleading. For example, in Pakistani-heritage languages, some actions are expressed as composite verb phrase consisting of a noun and a generic action, or "dummy do," component.

**Table 5.5** Example of errors in home language – omission

| Adult home-language utterance: *Target sentence* | kʊɾi | ɪʃaɾa | kaɾ-ni | pi |
|---|---|---|---|---|
| **Translation:** *morpheme-by-morpheme direct translation* | girl | point | doing + female | is + female |
| **Target translation:** *Best analogue in English/Mainstream language* | *(the) girl (she) is pointing* | | | |
| **Child/Young person's utterance:** *Transliterated verbatim in roman letters* | **"ishara kar-na"** | | | |
| **Morpheme-by-morpheme translation:** *Best analogue in English/Mainstream language preserving home language word/phrase order* | point do-ing + male | | | |
| **Closest English translation:** *Best analogue in English/Mainstream language using English/Mainstream language syntax and grammar* | (he) pointing | | | |
| **Clinician's comments:** *Differentiation between an acceptable synonym, different way of expressing the target utterance, and obvious errors and omissions which would not be acceptable to a home language-speaking adult* | • Omission of AGENT (Acceptable ellipsis or pattern in the data?)<br>• Omission of the auxiliary | | | |

**Table 5.6** Example of a composite verb phrase – noun + "dummy do"

| Adult home language utterance: *Target sentence* | kʊɾi | ɪʃaɾa | kaɾ-ni | pi |
|---|---|---|---|---|
| **Translation:** *morpheme-by-morpheme direct translation* | girl | point | doing + female | is + female |
| **Closest English translation:** *Best analogue in English/Mainstream language using English/Mainstream language syntax and grammar* | (the) girl is pointing | | | |

Note that in the Mirpuri utterance, "ishara" is not a verb, but rather a noun. The utterance is literally "the girl is doing a point." The "kar-" component is a "dummy do" component which allows the speaker to maintain the gender agreement (in this case female, as the agent is a girl).

Similarly, the Mirpuri language has another "dummy do" functioning as a *Noun + DO = ACTION* construction:

**Table 5.7** Example of a composite verb phrase – noun + "dummy do" with contact

| **Adult home-language utterance:**<br>*Target sentence* | d͡ʒənani | ʈaɾi | maɾ-ni | pi |
|---|---|---|---|---|
| **Translation:**<br>*morpheme-by-morpheme direct translation* | lady | clap | doing + female | is + female |
| **Closest English translation:**<br>*Best analogue in English/Mainstream language using English/Mainstream language syntax and grammar* | (the) lady/woman is clapping | | | |

In the example above, "mar-" is the "dummy do" component. Unlike, "kar-" in the previous example, "mar-" also encodes for *contact*. In this case, the woman's hands are making contact in the act of clapping. We see "mar-" employed for other verbs where contact is involved, including *brushing* (bəɾʌʃ / t͡ʃaɾu mar-na); *hopping* (t͡ʃal mar-na); *kicking* (qɪq mar-na)

As Mirpuri (and similarly Punjabi and Urdu) have been in contact with English in the UK for many decades, codeswitching into these structures is commonly encountered, with English verbs integrated as (underspecified) nouns.

In an assessment of 167 typically developing Pakistani-heritage Mirpuri, Punjabi, and Urdu speakers aged 2.6–7.2 years, 26 uninflected English verb stems were incorporated into compound verb phrases. These included "brush mar-ni"; "clap mar-ni"; "colour kar-ni"; "hoover mar-ni" (to vacuum clean; "Hoover" is a brand name often used as a verb in the UK, that is, "to hoover"); "climb kar-"; "throw kar-"; "smile kar-ni"; "draw kar-ni"; "sleep kar-na"; "clean kar-ni"; "make kar-ni"; "point kar-ni"; "smell kar-na"; "bath kar-na"; "walk kar-na" (Pert, 2007).

Similar examples have been found in Turkish/Dutch; Turkish/Norwegian (Myers-Scotton, 2002); English/Japanese (Azuma, 1993); English/Panjabi (Romaine, 1986); English/Panjabi (Martin et al., 2003); and English/Hindi (Grosjean, 1982).

Speech and language therapists should therefore treat codeswitching, especially where it matches home-language structures, as typical and normal language usage.

## Setting therapy aims – simple utterances

As seen above, English is relatively morphologically simple compared with many other languages. Aspects such as natural gender agreement, changing adjectives to match the gender of a noun, and other grammatical aspects may be unfamiliar to monolingual English-speaking speech and language therapists.

However, if these aspects are overlooked, then the child's progress is likely to be hampered. For goal/aim/target setting, there are some principles which may assist the professional working with a family with whom they do not share a language:

- Work alongside the interpreter/bilingual co-worker/bilingual speech and language therapy assistant to plan therapy aims
- Co-production: Involve the family. Are there particular activities where the child cannot get his meaning across that they would value working on at this time?
- Co-production: Involve the child or young person. Which home language activities do they enjoy and would like to be able to talk about more confidently?

Expressive language programmes where toy play, shared attention, signing morphological aspects and providing contrast and similarity across utterances have been shown to be effective in home language as well as English (McKean et al., 2010, 2013; Pert, 2011; Pert et al., 2014).

## Summary

Speech and language therapists must preserve the spoken language used by children and young people in their case notes. This is important for first comparison to evaluate any progress over time. In order to do this with service users from multiple language communities (and those bilingual communities where codeswitching is frequently employed), transliteration using the Roman alphabet is recommended as a universal notation accessible by the team.

Translation, even for simple spoken utterances is complex and involves cultural as well as linguistic knowledge. It is this process, identifying acceptable differences from errors and omissions which must be discussed with the interpreter after the language sample has been recorded. This is time-consuming and this is another reason why appointments with bilingual families should be at least double the time of that working with families with whom the therapist shares a language. Discussions during the de-brief should then lead to the comments in the translation protocol, as well as identifying patterns of errors and omissions which would make suitable targets/aims for therapy.

# References

Azuma, S. (1993). The frame-content hypothesis in speech production: Evidence from intrasentential code switching. *Linguistics, 31*, 1071–1093. https://doi.org/10.1515/ling.1993.31.6.1071.

Crystal, D. (1988). *Rediscover grammar with David Crystal.* Longman Group Limited.

Grosjean, F. (1982). *Life with two languages: An introduction to bilingualism.* Harvard University Press.

International Phonetic Association. (2015). *International phonetic alphabet.* www.internationalpho neticassociation.org/content/full-ipa-chart

Jaspal, R., & Coyle, A. (2010). "Arabic is the language of the Muslims-that's how it was supposed to be": Exploring language and religious identity through reflective accounts from young British-born South Asians. *Mental Health, Religion & Culture, 13*, 17–36. https://doi.org/10.1080/13674670903127205

Martin, D., Krishnamurthy, R., Bhardwaj, M., & Charles, R. (2003). Language change in young Panjabi/English children: Implications for bilingual language assessment. *Child Language Teaching and Therapy, 19*(3), 245–265.

McKean, C., Pert, S., & Stow, C. (2010). *Building early language patterns: Successful sentences in your language.* Royal College of Speech and Language Therapists' AGM and Study Day. www.research. manchester.ac.uk/portal/en/publications/building-early-language-patterns(f6157cbb-80b5-4319-b929-99b595083d94).html

McKean, C., Pert, S., & Stow, C. (2013). *Building Early Sentences Therapy (BEST) manual.* Newcastle University. https://www.research.ncl.ac.uk/media/sites/researchwebsites/languageinterventionin theearlyyears/BEST_Manual.pdf

Merriam-Webster. (2022). *Transliterate. Merriam-Webster.com dictionary.* Retrieved February 12, 2022, from www.merriam-webster.com/dictionary/transliterate

Myers-Scotton, C. (2002). *Contact Linguistics: Bilingual encounters and grammatical outcomes.* Oxford University Press. https://doi.org/10.1093/acprof:oso/9780198299530.001.0001

Pert, S. (2007). *Bilingual language development in Pakistani heritage children in Rochdale UK: Intrasentential codeswitching and the implications for identifying specific language impairment.* Newcastle University. http://www.theses.ncl.ac.uk/jspui/handle/10443/2230

Pert, S. (2011). *Building Early Sentences (BESt): Designing bilingual language interventions.* NALDIC. The Clothworkers' Centenary Concert Hall: The University of Leeds. www.research.manchester.ac.uk/ portal/en/publications/buidling-early-sentences-best(ccd9df2c-ba56-4004-b63d-e9ad107 89215).html

Pert, S., & Stow, C. J. (2002, January 14). *Mind the gap! Towards a translation protocol for speech and language therapists.* Royal College of Speech and Language Therapists' Special Interest Group in Bilingualism.

Pert, S., & Stow, C. J. (2003). *A translation protocol for speech and language therapists.* 5th CPLOL Conference. www.research.manchester.ac.uk/portal/en/publications/a-traceable-translation-proto col-for-speech-and-language-therapy-teams-working-with-bilingual-clients(89991c4f-9f91-4da5-90db-c9fa8e1ef5cf).html

Pert, S., Stow, C. J., & McKean, C. (2014). Building Early Sentences Therapy (BEST): Developing a theoretically driven, outcomes-focused therapy by involving practitioners, children and parents to maximise accessibility and acceptability. In *Royal college of speech and language therapists' conference 2014: Mind the gap: Putting research into practice.* University of Leeds. www.research.manches ter.ac.uk/portal/en/publications/building-early-sentences-therapy-best(67afde6f-8e59-4ca2-930d-088690a2fa38).html

Romaine, S. (1986). The syntax and semantics of the code-mixed compound verb in Panjabi/English bilingual discourse. In D. Tannen & J. E. Alatis (Eds.), *Languages and linguistics: The interdependence of theory, data and application.* Georgetown University Press.

Roulstone, S., Wren, Y., Bakopoulou, I., Goodlad, S., & Lindsay, G. (2012). *Exploring interventions for children and young people with speech, language and communication needs: A study of practice.* Department for Education. https://www.assets.publishing.service.gov.uk/government/uploads/sys tem/uploads/attachment_data/file/219627/DFE-RR247-BCRP13.pdf

Stow, C., Pert, S., & Khattab, G. (2012). Translation to practice: Sociolinguistic and cultural considerations when working with the Pakistani Heritage Community in England, UK. In S. Mcleod & B. A. Goldstein (Eds.), *Multilingual aspects of speech sound disorders in children.* Multilingual Matters.

# LANGUAGE ASSESSMENT AND INTERVENTION IN HOME LANGUAGE

DOI: 10.4324/9781003125563-6

## Which language(s) to assess and provide intervention?

Examples of scenarios are presented below. They are, of course, simplistic and the SLT will need to discuss both the desired outcome by adulthood ("Which languages do you wish your child to be able to speak when they are grown up?) and how committed parents are to the appropriate family language policy.

Successful language acquisition requires:

- Rich and well-formed language input from the parent(s)/carer (input of language data)
- Daily/very frequent use with activities of daily life carried out in that language (pragmatic aspects driving the need to acquire the language and shared attention)
- Conversational partners in that language who wish to, or need to converse in that language (social opportunities for interaction)

The following scenarios highlight the risks of linguistic isolation from one or both parents. This is the worst possible outcome for the child or young person. Cultural isolation, even for young people is potentially damaging to their sense of identity, mental health, and wellbeing. This may not be appreciated by the child or young person until they are well into adulthood.

Where parents/carers do not wish to follow the advice to use home language, then the high risk of language attrition should be documented in any reports and the case notes. When abandoning home language, parent(s) and carers should only do so when they are fully informed of the outcomes and risks.

I have encountered several families who did not believe that a mainstream approach would inevitability lead to the loss of the home language. Once the child has overcome their speech and/or language disorder, the family may then switch back to home language or provide language lessons. The drawback to this is that the child is likely to use English phonology and thus speak their parents' language with an English accent. Had they acquired both languages as a child it is likely that they will sound like a native speaker of both.

## Case illustration – abandoning home language due to Speech Sound Disorder

I recall an Urdu-English speaking mother rejecting home language intervention for her daughter aged 4;5 years and opting for an English-only approach. I wrote about the high risk of language attrition and loss in the report I provided after the initial assessment. The child was duly transferred to a monolingual English SLT who provided intervention in English only. The child overcame her Speech Sound Disorder, but lost her home language (Urdu), as her family language policy shifted to an English only one.

The child was re-referred to the Bilingual Service a few years later. Her mother complained that her daughter spoke "like an English girl trying to speak Urdu." The child in question did indeed replace retroflex phones with alveolar, fail to differentiate aspirated from unaspirated voiceless plosives, and make other typical errors an English speaker might make when attempting Urdu. The mother requested intervention in Urdu to remedy this.

The girl had acquired English and English phonology perfectly. I highlighted my written advice on the high risk of home-language attrition and loss. I declined the request to teach the child Urdu. This would have been additional language learning and therefore beyond the remit of the role of the SLT.

## Case illustration – abandoning home language due to language disorder

Punjabi speaking parents of a child aged 3.4 referred their son as he had failed to progress beyond single-word utterances. In common with many people in the community, there was a great deal of codeswitching in the parents' expressive language, and so the child had a range of Punjabi words, borrowings (words which have become part of Punjabi-English speakers' vocabulary and been integrated phonologically into Punjabi, such as "shopper" for shopping bag, pronounced ['ʃɒ.peɾ]), and English words such as "teddy."

The child's father spoke English well because he worked as a taxi driver, as well as fluent Punjabi. The child's mother had very basic English and spoke fluent Punjabi. The parents were very keen for their child to do well academically and so had begun to abandon their home language and speak only English. As the mother was the main carer, the child received English that was an incomplete model for language acquisition.

His parents insisted on an English-only intervention approach. The child went on to have pervasive difficulties with his language skills and was unable to speak Punjabi. This meant he was unable to speak to grandparents and the wider extended family. The child's relationship with his mother was hampered by the fact that his mother could not easily converse in English.

## Why not have a bilingual approach to intervention?

For languages that have equal status in a particular society, then a bilingual approach may well be possible. Some languages which were previously on the point of being lost have been revived. Examples include Welsh and Māori. It is notable that both of these examples have cultures where the languages are supported by increasing social status and home-language education. However, for most bilingual speakers, especially those speaking languages originating from outside of Europe, this is often not the case.

Many children and young people will only gain experience of home languages in the home environment. It is also important to consider that exposure to the mainstream language in education is sufficient to acquire that language.

"Even if (mothers) have really, really poor English language skills, they're trying to teach their child in English because they think that's what the education system wants them to do, and what I used to spend a lot of time doing is encouraging parents that at home you speak the language that you are fluent and good at. Because then you're giving your child that good foundation. And school will deal with the English and you can work with both together so at home or speech and language therapy we can work in the mother tongue and we can build that up and in the school environment their English will build and we can build both up together."

*Zahida Warriach, Senior Bilingual Speech and Language Therapy*
*Assistant, mother of bilingual children and multilingual speaker.*

Delivering one-to-one or group therapy in the mainstream language (typically English) will halve the time spend on the home language. Literacy may not be an option to develop home language skills, especially if the language is preliterate. The home language needs as much support as possible as only family and the local community can provide input.

The child will hear mainstream input from friends at school, older siblings, and their teacher; in pop music, films (movies), and television programmes; and through literacy. These high-status and highly motivating sources mean that the mainstream language rarely needs the same level of support as the home language. The mainstream language is also not at risk of attrition since the child or young person encounters it in school, shops, and the wider world.

**Table 6.1** Illustrations of the language of assessment and intervention and advice

| Child | Home situation | Attitude of parent(s)/carer to home language | Language usage by the child | Advice from SLT | Language of assessment and intervention | Points to consider |
|---|---|---|---|---|---|---|
| Pre-school 0–4 years of age Sequential bilingual/ Monolingual in a language other than English Suspected language disorder Single words, or limited expressive language | One or both parent(s)/carer only speaks home language or has minimal skills in the additional/ mainstream language | Wish child to speak the mainstream language/ language of education as concerned home language will hold back the child and/or home language has caused speech and/or language disorder | Home language | Debunk myths of home language slowing down the acquisition of mainstream language (such as English) and that home language use caused the speech/language disorder | Home language An interpreter is required. | If parent(s)/carer use their limited mainstream language this will provide a poor model for language acquisition for young children Mainstream language approach is likely to isolate the child from their immediate carer(s) |
| Pre-school 0–4 years of age Sequential bilingual/ Monolingual in a language other than English Suspected language disorder Single words, or limited expressive language | Parents speak both home language and mainstream language to a high level Parents speak both home language and mainstream language to the child | Wish child to speak both languages | Home language and mainstream language | Switch family language policy to home language only, as this is the only source of the language Advise that mainstream language will be acquired through exposure in educational setting | Home language An interpreter is required | Mainstream language approach is likely to lead to a gradual language attrition of home language over several years Child likely to switch completely to the mainstream language on school entry, especially if home language is perceived as having a lower status than the home language. Warn parents that this is likely to happen and advise that when it does, they should still use their home language back to their child even if he uses the mainstream language to them.' |

*(Continued)*

**Table 6.1** (Continued)

| Child | Home situation | Attitude of parent(s)/carer to home language | Language usage by the child | Advice from SLT | Language of assessment and intervention | Points to consider |
|---|---|---|---|---|---|---|
| Pre-school 0–4 years of age Only hears and speaks English Suspected language disorder Single words, or limited expressive language | Parents/carers are bilingual but only speak English to the children | Wish the child to speak English only | English only | This is a monolingual English-speaking child. See "Points to consider." | Mainstream language (English) | If parent(s)/carers wish their child to speak home language, then they will need to change family language policy to home language only OR provide lessons for the language as a formal educational route in the future (child likely to have an English accent when speaking this language) |
| Key Stage 1 Foundation Year 1 Year 2 5–7 years old Sequential bilingual Suspected language disorder Limited expressive language | One or both parent(s)/carer only speaks home language or has minimal skills in the additional/ mainstream language. | Concerned that child is not doing well academically at school. Wishes the child to use the mainstream language well. | Uses mainly mainstream language (English) at home, even though mother has no/limited skills. Speaks English at school. | Opportunity to acquire the home language in the early years was lost due to language disorder. Recommend a language policy of home language only to restore/ develop home language skills. | Home language and Mainstream languages for assessment Home language for intervention An interpreter is required | Even if the child has no home-language skills, the potential damage from continuing on a monolingual mainstream language approach is likely to isolate the child from his mother. Risks to mental health and wellbeing, as well as cultural isolation in the future. The child may object to the switch to home language for several months. This is typically expressed by speaking only English, and/or commenting that they don't want to talk differently to their peers. |

| | | | | | | |
|---|---|---|---|---|---|---|
| Key Stage 1 Foundation Year 1 Year 2 5–7 years old Sequential bilingual Suspected language disorder Limited expressive language | Parents speak both home language and mainstream language to a high level. Parents speak both home language and mainstream language to the child. | Concerned that child is not doing well academically at school Wishes the child to use the mainstream language well | Uses mainly mainstream language (English) at home. When mother uses home language the child replies in the mainstream language (English) Speaks the mainstream language (English) at school | Opportunity to acquire the home language in the early years was lost due to language disorder Recommend a language policy of home language only | Home language and Mainstream languages for assessment Home language for intervention An interpreter is required | Use of a mainstream only approach will lead to an increase in mainstream language until home language is eliminated/lost to attrition. Risks to mental health and wellbeing, as well as cultural isolation in the future The child may object to the switch to home language for several months |
| Key Stage 2 Year 3–6 8–11 years old Sequential bilingual Suspected language disorder Expressive language affected | One or both parent(s)/carer only speaks home language or has minimal skills in the additional/ mainstream language | Concerned that child is not doing well academically at school Wishes the child to use the mainstream language well | Uses mainly mainstream language (English) at home, even though mother has no/limited skills Has some receptive language skills Very limited home language expression Speaks English at school | Opportunity to acquire the home language in the early years was lost due to language disorder Recommend formal home language lessons for the child if available Recommend mainstream language lessons for parent(s) Aim to facilitate good communication between parents and child | Home language and Mainstream languages for assessment An interpreter is required Mainstream language for intervention | There is already a process of isolation between parent(s) and child which needs urgent attention The child cannot acquire the home language and requires formal lessons in home language An interpreter is still required to support the parent(s) |

*(Continued)*

**Table 6.1** (Continued)

| Child | Home situation | Attitude of parent(s)/carer to home language | Language usage by the child | Advice from SLT | Language of assessment and intervention | Points to consider |
|---|---|---|---|---|---|---|
| Key Stage 2 Year 3–6 8–11 years old Sequential bilingual Suspected language disorder Expressive language affected | Parents speak both home language and mainstream language to a high level Parents speak both home language and mainstream language to the child | Concerned that child is not doing well academically at school Wishes the child to use the mainstream language well | Uses mainly mainstream language (English) at home. When mother uses home language the child replies in the mainstream language (English) Speaks the mainstream language (English) at school | Opportunity to acquire the home language in the early years was lost due to language disorder Recommend a language policy of home language only | Home language and Mainstream languages for assessment Home language for intervention An interpreter is required. | The parents are well-placed to help their child to use and value home language. They can re-phrase any English expression at home into home language Parents may need reassurance that a home language only family language policy will not affect the child's educational performance The child may object to the switch to home language for several months |
| Key Stage 3 onwards Year 7–13 12–18 years old Sequential bilingual Suspected language disorder Expressive language affected | One or both parent(s)/carer only speaks home language or has minimal skills in the additional/ mainstream language | Concerned that child is not doing well academically at school Wishes the child to use the mainstream language well | Uses mainly mainstream language (English) at home, even though mother has no/limited skills Has some, or no receptive language skills in home language No/very limited home language expression Speaks English at school | Opportunity to acquire the home language in the early years was lost due to language disorder Recommend formal home language lessons for the child if available Recommend mainstream language lessons for parent(s) Aim to facilitate good communication between parents and child | Mainstream language for assessment Mainstream language for intervention | The process of linguistic isolation between parent(s) and child is complete The child will need formal lessons in home language if they are to develop expressive skills in that language. An interpreter is still required to support the parent(s) |

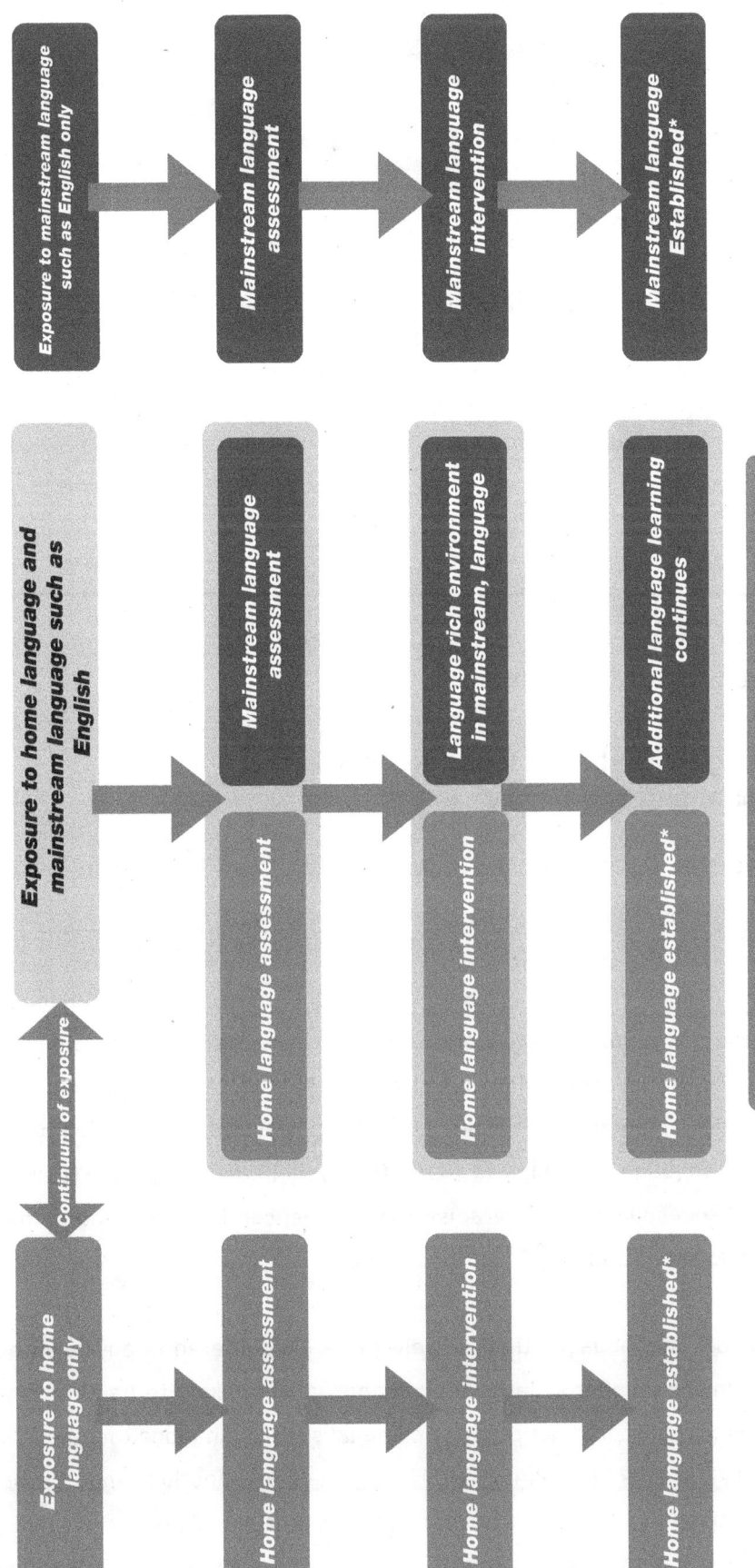

**Figure 6.1** Which language for assessment and intervention

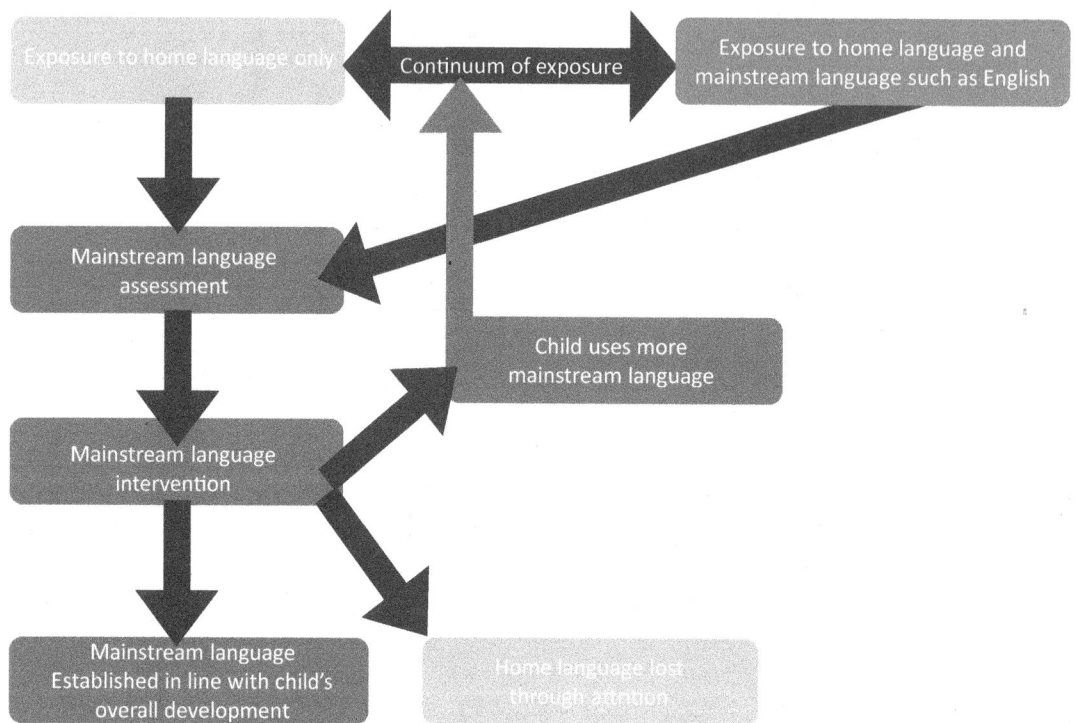

**Figure 6.2** Home language attrition model

## Shared language/NO shared language between the professional and the family

This chapter discusses working in home language when there is NO shared language between the SLT and the family or client.

It should be acknowledged that there are a growing number of bilingual/multi-lingual SLTs who obviously have the opportunity to work with more than one language community. If the SLT has a near native level of proficiency, then they need not work alongside an interpreter for that particular language community. It is the professional responsibility of each SLT or professional to judge her ability to work effectively in that language. Therefore, if you are a bilingual speech language therapist and you feel confident working in that language you should go ahead and do so.

However, the number of languages that is likely to be encountered in any town or city is much larger than the number of languages an individual is likely to be able to speak with this level of proficiency. In practice, most bilingual speech language therapists speak English (as it is likely that they qualified in this language), and another language or two. Most towns and cities have communities that speak tens if not hundreds of languages. A bilingual SLT who spoke for example English, French and Italian would still need to work alongside an interpreter in order to work with families from other language communities.

This is why working alongside an interpreter is a core skill for all SLTs, whether monolingual English or bilingual (Royal College of Speech and Language Therapists, 2021).

## Interpreter or bilingual SLT?

There will never be sufficient SLTs who speak all the languages encountered on a typical caseload. The default way of working should be to work alongside an interpreter who speaks the home language of the client and family, and the SLT.

There are, of course, bilingual SLTs. These professionals can work with their language communities but will still need to work with interpreters when working with speakers of other languages.

## When the shared language is not the home language

Many bilingual families have skills in a set of languages due to educational exposure, the political situation in their home country, or experiences of living in one country prior to settling in another country.

Invasion, political interference, religious missions, and colonialism by European powers across Africa, India, and America have left a legacy of education and European languages spoken across the world. These languages, such as Spanish, English, French, and Portuguese, may evolve into their own unique variants. In other communities, they may sit alongside the home language, often as the language of education. Access to these colonial education systems was (and often still is) limited by race and gender (Griffiths, 2008).

If a family speaks a European language, this may be attractive as a lingua-franca. However, the use of a colonial language will ignore the family's home language. SLTs should aim to work in the home language, and not necessarily the language(s) of education. It may be convenient to communicate using a shared language such as French, but effort must be made to identify a home language interpreter. Reputable interpreter companies should be able to locate a home language speaker, even if this is only via telehealth.

## Assessing language skills

Assessing language skills is a core part of the routine initial assessment carried out by SLTs. For a language such as English, the child and the SLT often share a language. This means that the SLT can confidently adapt their questions and responses. This is especially important if the child cannot understand and the SLT has to move to simpler instructions, or if the child needs scaffolding and prompting to produce expressive language.

This "step down" in complexity and scaffolding and prompting cannot be delivered in the same spontaneous way when the child and the SLT do not share a language.

Instead, these must be pre-planned with the interpreter. Fortunately, this is not as complex as it first appears. This chapter will examine how to plan for assessment and identify possible cultural and linguistic pitfalls you may encounter.

## Assessing home language skills and then additional language skills

The pragmatics of assessment are a key consideration when undertaking an assessment of a bilingual child's speech and language skills. That is, the expectations and unspoken "rules" of communication settings and of the people we encounter.

Many bilingual children perceive educational settings as the place where **only** their additional language is spoken (typically English). This is because their teachers use English, their friends use English, and all learning activities are typically in this language.

The other pragmatic aspect is the perception of the people involved in assessment. In the UK, 93.4% of those SLTs surveyed reported that they were white. It is not possible to equate ethnicity with bilingualism. However, for children from Black, Asian, and minority ethnic backgrounds who do speak another language at home, they would be very surprised to meet a white professional who speaks their language.

In my own clinical practice, when I have spoken Mirpuri to a Pakistani-heritage child, they have often laughed and been greatly surprised as they have never before encountered a white man who spoke to them in their home language. Even for white bilingual children, they would often be reticent to use their home language, as they will have observed that others do not use their home language in such settings.

To overcome these strong pragmatic signals that their home language will not be welcome, SLTs must ensure that home language is used from the start of the session. This may include using telehealth or carrying out a home visit (since the pragmatics for using a home language will be very strong for the home setting). The extended family may also be in the home setting and encourage the child to use home language in the course of their everyday interactions. If the appointment is in a clinical setting, asking the interpreter to greet the family in home language, and using a few words yourself will signal that home language is acceptable in this setting (Stow et al., 2012). Just as when working with any child who is new to an environment, "settling in" activities, such as free pretend play, small world toys or games, and conversations in home language, will also provide the signal that home language is appropriate and welcomed. It is important to have play materials that are familiar to the child and their culture, such as dolls wearing traditional clothing such as shalwar kameez, toy foods that reflect the child's diet, and images on the walls of people from different cultures.

It is useful to encourage the use of both/all language the child speaks, as codeswitching is normal in most bilingual communities. However, use of both languages may push the child back into using just the additional language. It is therefore helpful to assess home language and then have a break or play session prior to assessing the additional language. If there are lots of assessments and tasks it may be better to assess the additional language on another occasion and possibly in a different setting.

## Thematic roles

Thematic roles (Saeed, 2003, pp. 148–164) are thought to be universal to human language. Consider the English *subject*. In the utterance "the cat chases the mouse," the cat is the subject of the sentence. However, if we use a passive construction "the mouse is chased **by the cat**," then the mouse is now the subject of the sentence. The terms "subject," "verb," and "object" refer to the *surface structure* of English, not to the properties of the mouse or cat.

Thematic roles refer to the function of the different aspects of the utterance. These functions do not change with word/phrase order or surface form of a particular language, but are properties that humans understand.

In our example, the cat is always the "chaser," the one doing the action. This role, termed the **AGENT**, is taken by a person, animal, or entity that has volition and ability to undertake actions. The mouse is the thing undergoing the action carried out by the AGENT. The mouse is the **PATIENT**. The verb or **ACTION** is also important to consider in relation to surface form. In some languages the ACTION may be mapped to a single lexical verb, whilst in others in may be mapped to a "doing" generic verb and a noun. Contrasting surface forms for some familiar verbs are listed in Table 6.2.

**Table 6.2** Thematic roles

| THEMATIC ROLE | DESCRIPTION |
| --- | --- |
| AGENT | the "doer"; "the initiator of some action, capable of acting with volition" |
| PATIENT | the "done to"; "the entity undergoing the effect of some action, often undergoing some change in state" |
| ACTION (VERB) | this sets the relationship between the other thematic roles |
| THEME | "the entity moved by an action, or whose location is described" |
| EXPERIENCER | "the entity which is aware of the action or state described by the predicate but which is not in control of the action or state" |
| BENEFICIARY | "the entity for whose benefit the action was performed" |
| INSTRUMENT | "the means by which an action is performed or something comes about" |
| LOCATION | "the place in which something is situated or takes place" |
| GOAL | "the entity towards which something moves, either literally . . . or metaphorically" |
| SOURCE | "the entity from which something moves, either literally . . . or metaphorically" |

Adapted from Saeed (2003, pp. 148–180).

**Table 6.3** Surface structure versus thematic roles

| Utterance | the cat | chased | the mouse |
| --- | --- | --- | --- |
| Thematic roles | AGENT "the chaser" | ACTION | PATIENT "the one chased" |
| Surface form | Subject | Verb | Object |
| Utterance | the mouse | is chased | by the cat |
| Thematic roles | PATIENT "the one chased" | ACTION | AGENT "the chaser" |

Note how the thematic roles are unchanged, regardless of surface structure.

**Table 6.4** Examples of verbs where English and Mirpuri languages contrast on surface argument structure

| Example 1: "hopping" or "doing a hop" | | |
| --- | --- | --- |
| ENGLISH utterance | the girl | is hopping |
| Thematic roles | AGENT | ACTION |
| Surface form | Subject | Verb |
| Phrase | Noun Phrase | Verb Phrase |
| Mapping | determiner + head noun | auxiliary + lexical verb-present progressive morpheme |
| MIRPURI utterance | kuri | chal mar-ni pi |
| | | • *jump (noun)* |
| | | • *do (with contact)-present progressive+ female agreement with subject "girl"* |
| | | • *auxiliary is + female agreement with subject "girl"* |
| Thematic roles | AGENT | ACTION |
| Surface form | Subject | Verb |
| Phrase | Noun Phrase | Verb Phrase |
| Mapping | head noun | noun + generic doing verb + contact (with the floor) |
| | | Literally "doing a hop" |
| Comments | English maps the ACTION onto a **lexical verb** which is intransitive | Mirpuri maps the ACTION onto a **compound verb phrase that includes a noun** and a generic "dummy do." |

Example 2: "pointing" or "doing a point"

| | | |
|---|---|---|
| ENGLISH utterance | the girl | is pointing |
| Thematic roles | AGENT | ACTION |
| Surface form | Subject | Verb |
| Phrase | Noun Phrase | Verb Phrase |
| Mapping | determiner + head noun | auxiliary + lexical verb-present progressive morpheme |
| MIRPURI utterance | kuri | ishara kar-ni pi |
| | | • *point (noun) +* |
| | | • *do -present progressive-female agreement with subject "girl"* |
| | | • *auxiliary is + female agreement with subject "girl"* |
| Thematic roles | AGENT | ACTION |
| Surface form | Subject | Verb |
| Phrase | Noun Phrase | Verb Phrase |
| Mapping | head noun | noun + generic doing verb |
| | | Literally "doing a point" |
| Comments | English maps the ACTION onto a **lexical verb** which is intransitive | Mirpuri maps the ACTION onto a **compound verb phrase that includes a noun** and a generic "dummy do" |

## Using thematic roles to analyse bilingual utterances

Bilingual children with language disorder are likely to have problems at one or more levels of mapping meaning to spoken utterance surface forms. This will affect both/all the languages that they speak. To examine the level of breakdown, just as we might with speech sound production, it is important to consider where the child is experiencing difficulties. The "deeper" the difficulty, the more likely this will have a knock-on effect to more surface structures.

## Usage-based language acquisition

Human children are able to speak the language(s) that they are exposed to. As Tomasello (2003, p. 1) highlights, "Young children must learn . . . the set of linguistic conventions used by those around them, which for any given language consists of tens of thousands, or perhaps even hundreds of thousands, of individual words, expressions, and constructions."

For the child exposed to two or more language codes, this poses a much bigger task than acquiring just one language. This is one of the reasons that bilingual children, from the perspective of the monolingual, appear to be "delayed." This unfair comparison with the monolingual child is patently unfair and fails to consider the child's language skills holistically.

For very young children in the earliest stages of language acquisition, comprehension will tend to exceed expression. This is partly due to the fact that speech requires *physical* fine-motor control, which young children are still in the process of developing.

**Table 6.5** Analysis of errors for a Mirpuri simple utterance

| *Mirpuri target utterance:* | *mura* | *kela* | *kha-na pi-ja* |
|---|---|---|---|
| *Morpheme-by- morpheme translation* | *boy* | *banana* | *eat-ing + male is + male* |
| *Nearest English equivalent:* | *(the) boy (he) is eating* | | |

| Level of difficulty | Surface pattern examples | Examples |
|---|---|---|
| Thematic roles not developed | No verbal output<br>Gross errors on syntax<br>Omits one or more phrases*<br>Single-word naming (nouns) | "mura"<br>*boy*<br>"mura kela"<br>*boy banana* |
| Mapping from thematic roles to surface form | Relationships between AGENTS and PATIENTS not signalled, or<br>AGENT repeated as patient phrase (not a fluency issue, but a content repeated insertion into the utterance frame)<br>ACTIONS under specified/omitted | "mura kha-na"<br>*boy eat-ing + male*<br>"kela kela khan-na"<br>*banana banana eat-ing + male*<br>"mura kar-na"<br>*boy do-ing + male* |
| Between phrase errors | Gender agreement with AGENTS (if part of the language) omitted or only one form used, such as the male form for all examples | "mura kela kha-na"<br>*boy banana eat-ing + male*<br>*"kuri kela kha-na"<br>*girl banana eat-ing + male*<br>*instead of*<br>"kuri kela kha-ni" |
| Within phrase errors | Determiners (if part of the language) omitted and/or gender/number agreement errors<br>Verb tense errors/omissions<br>Auxiliary verb errors/omissions | "mura khela kha-na"<br>*omitted auxiliary utterance-final "pi-ja" (is + male)* |
| Content word errors/ codeswitching not used or errors made | Unable to integrate home language into additional language and maintain phrase/word order and essential morphology of the morphosyntactic frame language | Avoids codeswitching.<br>Poor verb-agreement/ morphology. |

Complex psycholinguistic processes are used to "break the code" of the language(s) they are exposed to. Language structures (syntax, grammar, and morphology) are abstracted from the language that children hear around them together with the activities and events that they observe or take part in.

This learning is facilitated by **shared attention** with other speakers. Children hear language paired with an object and/or action and map that language by comparing with their previous knowledge and experience. So, for example, if a parent says "Look! the dog's running!" and the child already knows the word "dog" from previous learning, then they will be more likely to map the word "run" as the action. They will be able to **compare and contrast** with other events, such as the parent commenting on other people and animals running to confirm their hypothesis. The presence of "-ing" will be compared with other action words. In this way, the child learns language through experiences shared with others. The child reads the **intentions** of the adult speaker to highlight the event (See Ambridge & Lieven, 2011 for a full discussion of theories of child language acquisition).

Why is the theory of language acquisition important? The vast majority of language therapy focuses on *surface structures*, and on the English language, since most SLTs are English monolingual speakers. If the clinician can understand and apply a universal model of language acquisition, then this should be applicable to all speakers, with attention paid to the common processes, as well as the surface projection of the language onto a spoken utterance.

The *Building Early Sentences Therapy* (BEST) (McKean et al., 2013a) applies these principles to both monolingual English speakers, speakers of languages other than English (LOTE) and speakers of two or more languages (bilingual children) who are experiencing language disorder. The therapy package does not treat language as a tower, with more complex language structures built on top of simpler structures (in a way that more complex utterances *rely* on establishing more simple ones), but rather exposes the child to actions using toys, along with spoken utterances. Children are sometimes able to acquire "harder" sentence structures before "easier" ones, such as prepositional phrases prior to simple AGENT+ACTION+PATIENT (*subject + verb + object surface form for English*) utterances, or, of course AGENT+PATIENT+ACTION (*subject + object + verb surface form in Mirpuri*).

The therapy involves providing utterances that are organised so as to provide variation and contrast with distributed sentence patterns. This helps the child to abstract the language rules and use that language themselves.

The important aspect to note, is that comprehension of language arises not as a discrete process to expression. Children often use utterances they do not completely understand, but in using them, they observe the actions and this feeds into their understanding. This cycle of "use language ➜ observe the effect ➜ update understanding" challenges the traditional therapy model of "comprehension precedes expression." This means that clinicians can, in most cases focus on input-based therapy and not insist that children *demonstrate* understanding prior to moving onto expression.

This phenomenon of expression exceeding comprehension is also observed in typically developing children. For example, Hendriks and Spenader (2005) found that children made errors on comprehending pronouns as late as 6 years 6 months yet used them correctly from age 2 or 3 years.

## Verbal comprehension

As discussed, it is unlikely for most children and young people that comprehension and expression will be affected separately in bilingual children with language disorder. Broomfield and Dodd (2004) found that "expressive language and vocabulary difficulties co-occurred for virtually all children with comprehension disability." It is therefore important to assess language skills as a whole.

There are very few published assessments of verbal comprehension in languages other than English. Adaptation of assessments available in English is complex and will require the collation of new normative data on bilingual children since the normative data will be available for children who have only ever spoken English. This is beyond the remit and capability of most individual practitioners and services.

If assessment of verbal comprehension is required separately from expression, then care must be taken to ensure that cultural, pragmatic and linguistic barriers are not inadvertently placed in the way of the child succeeding in such tasks.

Children may not recognise objects, activities, food and drink that is featured in most published materials. Many children are unused to adults interacting with them, especially in their home language, and may refuse to respond due to the unfamiliarity of the testing situation. Translating requested may also have pitfalls, as languages rarely have the same subtle meanings. For example, "Show me the OBJECT" in Mirpuri may not a typical activity for parents and children, and the translation of this seemingly simple instruction may have more in common with "Display the OBJECT."

A simple verb such as "waving" can be problematic for both linguistic and cultural reasons. Many parents reported that children are taught to clap, and that waving is not expected in very young children. The translation of "waving" offered is shown in Table 6.6.

**Table 6.6** Example of a lexical verb not known in a language: "waving"

| Mirpuri instruction | miki | das | bander | hat$^h$ hala-na |
|---|---|---|---|---|
| Morpheme-by-morpheme translation | me | show | monkey | hand move -ing + male |
| Nearest English equivalent | show me (the) monkey moving (his) hand | | | |
| | Nearest equivalent to "show me (the) monkey **waving**" | | | |

Clearly, this is not a single lexical verb, like "waving." The interpreter was trying to offer the closest translation. On discussion however, the decision to replace this item with a more culturally familiar item was taken ("clapping"). This reflects the different styles of language usage and interaction between English speaking and monolingual English-speaking communities.

As a result of these understandable differences in language, culture and pragmatics, it is important to discuss the familiarity of words, items and activities used in assessment with the interpreter *prior to seeing the client*. This should lead to an **adaptation** of the assessment materials, **never** a surface translation where these issues have not been considered.

For all these reasons, direct and detailed assessment of comprehension skills may not be possible using a single tool. Where possible, assessment of verbal comprehension should instead be carried out using parental interviews, observations in home and home language situations with other children, and informal assessment of concepts and instructions that are important to everyday interactions.

As it is easier to hear and analyse expressive language skills, it may be that it is assumed that if the child cannot use the language concept or structure, that they do not have full acquisition of it in terms of comprehension. Therapy aimed at improving the use of language will also facilitate comprehension. It is *not* essential for a child to understand a concept or instruction prior to commencing expressive language therapy. This obviously does *not* apply to children or young people where a physical disability, acquired language impairment or psychological condition such as selective mutism is present. If comprehension skills need to be assessed separately, then culturally and linguistically adapted versions of assessments may be devised. For example, the *New Reynell Language Developmental Language Scales* (NRDLS) (See Letts et al., 2014) includes a Multilingual Toolkit. Examples of adaptations of the NRDLS where scoring and complexity of instructions has been considered are now available in Polish and Sylheti (LIVELY, in press).

## Vocabulary and expressive language

The meaning of even single words is affected by translation. Take for example "bread," a noun (naming word). Is a "roti" (a flat bread made on a flat iron pan or griddle, "tawa" or "tava") the same as a loaf? Clearly not!

Translating even a verb can cause changes in morphology and even word number. In Mirpuri "jump" is a noun, not a verb. Therefore one "does a jump." The language also requires that

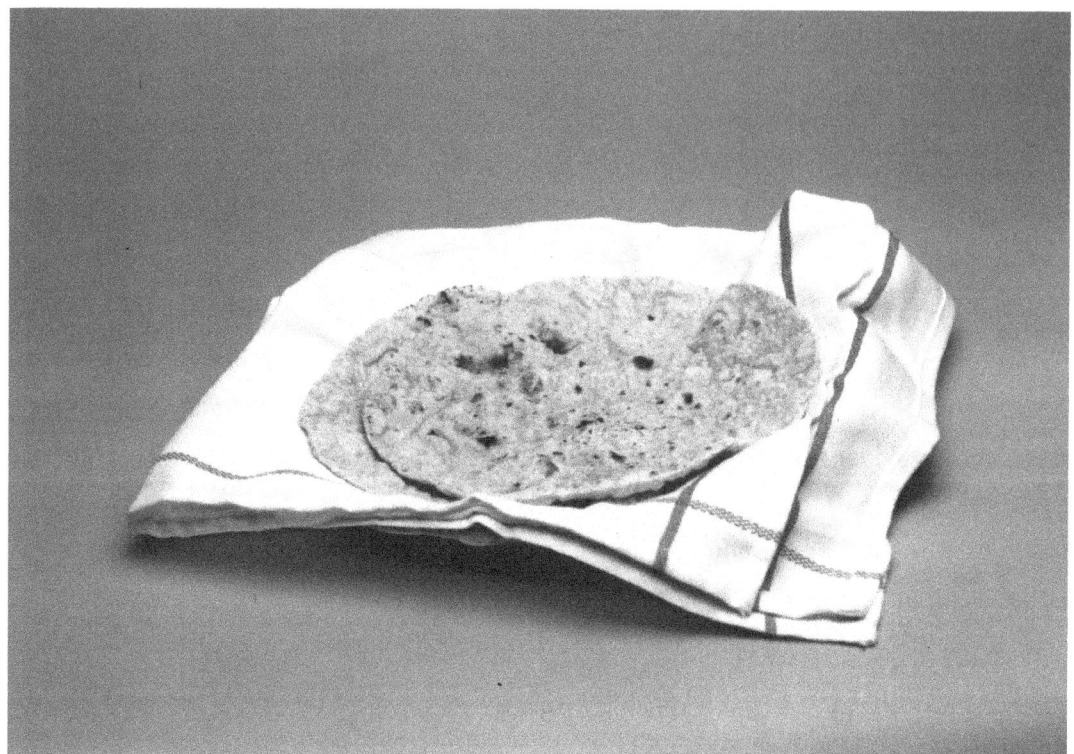

**Figure 6.3** Roti, a traditional Pakistani flatbread

the present progressive (-ing) agrees with the natural gender of the agent. So if a child says "kha-na," this literally means "eating + male" (i.e., a boy or man is eating). An interpreter might translate this as "He's eating" as the nearest English version. However, the child did not use a pronoun or an auxiliary (never mind a contracted auxiliary), and only used one word.

Some items may be different across communities, or unknown in one community but commonplace in another. Examples of differences between the Pakistani-heritage community and the white monolingual community include food items. "Bengan" are small aubergines found in community stores. Larger sized ones sold in supermarkets are seldom recognised by Pakistani heritage children. "Karela" (bitter gourd), a knobbly green vegetable that is frequently used in curry, is virtually unknown by white monolingual families.

This chapter will examine how to avoid these pitfalls with templates for identifying common nouns and alerting you to possible differences between languages. The use of the translation protocol (Pert & Stow, 2003) will make expressive language data collection simpler and more systematic.

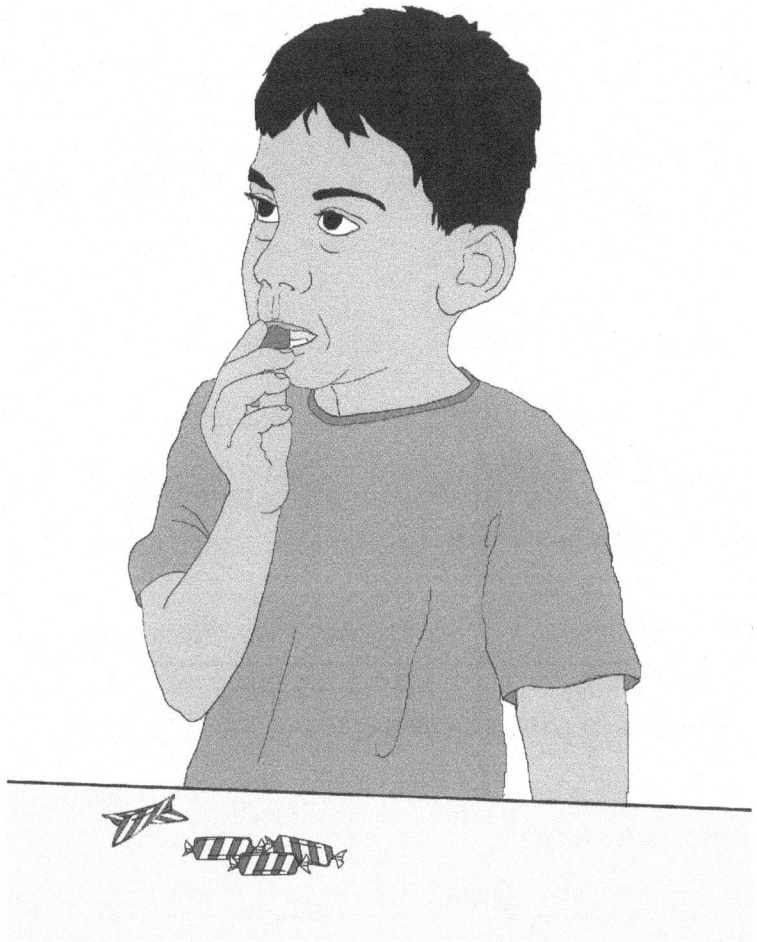

**Figure 6.4** The boy is eating

There may be a physical reason that speech cannot be produced, such as children with cerebral palsy or similar conditions. However, such children will be able to use language in the form of Augmentative and Alternative Communication (AAC) and/or signing systems. This is discussed in another chapter in this book.

## Comorbidity

Many children do not present with just one speech and language disorder. For example, it is very common for children with speech disorder to also have language disorder (Broomfield & Dodd, 2004; Eadie et al., 2015; Shriberg et al., 1999). This is important, as many language concepts are used in speech therapy, and therapy addressing speech sounds may fail because the child cannot yet use certain concepts such as "long"/"short" or "loud"/"quiet."

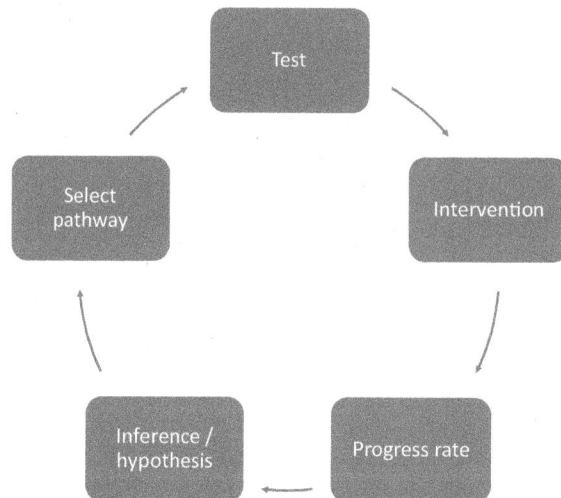

**Figure 6.5** Dynamic assessment model

For bilingual children, differential diagnosis is vital. Many professionals confuse additional language learning problems with a core speech and Language Difficulty. This section will examine how to differentiate difference from disorder.

## Pragmatic language skills

Different cultural norms exist, and this can be confusing if the SLT is only familiar with British English norms. For example, children from a Pakistani-heritage background may be expected to avoid eye contact with adults. This may be misinterpreted as a sign of social communication disorder or withdrawal.

Initiation, turn-taking and other rules of conversation may also differ.

Most importantly, bilingual children try to use the correct language for the person and setting they are in. For example, children quickly realise that English is spoken in school and may be reluctant to use their home language in that setting.

This section will examine how to make the child comfortable using home language in clinical situations and how to recognise cultural differences.

## Informal and formal assessments of language

Standardised and published formal assessments are often seen as "the gold standard" and as such are routinely used for the assessment of children's receptive and expressive language skills in English. In fact, most SLTs take formal assessments so much for granted that they overlook the limitations of these assessment tools even for monolingual English-speaking children. All of these assessments attempt to evaluate child's language ability in a convenient manner. No assessments can comprehensively address this complex task. However, most typically developing children are able to cope with these fairly unusual tasks.

While most English monolingual speaking children are familiar with books, carrying out instructions, and interacting with adults, this may not always be the case with children from other cultures. Some languages are pre-literate (have no written form) and so books may be unfamiliar.

Cultural difference can make a huge difference to how children and young people respond. I recall a case where a young traveller boy was referred to my service with concerns about his ability to use expressive language. Indeed, he was very quiet in clinic and found talking about pictures unusual. That was until I showed him a picture of a horse. Horses are central to traveller culture, especially to boys and young men where they represent not only the culture but also prestige and skill (Rowland et al., 2019). This young boy was able to provide me with copious detail about the care and training of horses. His sentences were well formed but contained variations from standard English. This is an example where the assessment materials failed to elicit an appropriate response not because the child did not have expressive language capability, but rather the stimulus materials did not match his life experience.

## Language screen versus detailed language assessment

A screen of any kind is a brief examination of the targeted skill. If the child or young person is able to effortlessly provide the appropriate response, then we move on to other aspects of assessment. It is not appropriate to reach a firm diagnosis using just a screen. Rather, a full evaluation of all areas within that particular domain should be undertaken. With standardised assessments this is often possible due to the many sections making up the full standardised test. For children who speak languages other than English, this is a big challenge. How can we assess all the areas of the child's language, making the subtests culturally and linguistically appropriate?

## Why informal home language assessments are superior to published standardised English language assessments

Although there are increasing numbers of publications providing normative data for both monolingual and bilingual acquisition of many languages we may encounter, there are no data or insufficient data for many languages and dialects. In reality therefore, it is not possible to replicate a comprehensive and detailed assessment of language using a series of informal assessments. However, informal assessments which attempt to include materials that are culturally appropriate, are far superior to any ad hoc adaption of a published standardised assessment. We must not lose sight of the fact that parents and carers and indeed the child or young person themselves will not value their home language and favour English if we deliver assessment entirely in English. Professionals have status and privilege and as such employing home language in assessment means that we are signalling that it is of central importance to the child's development and the family as a whole.

## Assessment of comprehension: early years

In the UK, the tradition is to assess verbal comprehension separately from expression through the ability to carry out instructions of increasing complexity using real objects, toys and pictures. English is relatively morphologically poor language (Avramidis & Koehn, 2008). When assessing morphologically rich languages, speakers of English may fail to consider the impact on the assessment of verbal comprehension skills.

For example, in Mirpuri, verbs and auxiliary verbs agree with the agent's natural gender (subject). One must therefore signal the gender in the question. It is therefore important to have pictures of children all of the same gender for this section of the assessment, or the question may give away the answer if the "washing" picture is the only one portraying a boy, while the others are girls carrying out actions.

Other examples of differences between English and Mirpuri include word/phrase order, which may be important for children with short term memory or processing difficulties, and specific grammatical and morphological differences, such as marking the location for prepositions.

Translation of assessment materials must also involve cultural adaptation, as children may fail to recognise an item simply because they do not encounter it in their everyday life. For Pakistani-heritage children, knives and forks are less familiar due to the use of *roti* (flat breads) for eating *salan* (curry).

There are translated and culturally adapted versions descriptive assessments such as the *Functional Language Across Countries* (FLAC) (Millar-Wilson, 2014) available in several

**Table 6.7** Example of a question with embedded gender

| kira | to-na | pi-ja |
| --- | --- | --- |
| which-one | wash-ing + male | is + male |
| Who's washing? | | |

languages. Such informal assessments attempt to accommodate cultural differences and deliver an assessment that will not diagnose a typically developing bilingual child as having Language Difficulties, simply because they don't recognise the test items, or worse are only assessed in their additional language.

Linguistic translation issues and cultural differences make it challenging to assess verbal comprehension, especially as translated and culturally adapted versions may not be available, or the time to develop such resources is not feasible. For such languages, parental report may be the best option, especially for pre-school children.

The MacArthur-Bates *Communicative Developmental Inventories* (CDIs) have been adapted (not simply translated) to meet the needs of several different speech communities (Dale, 2015).

**Table 6.8** Recommendations for assessing language skills – checklist

| | **Assess home language skills first in a single session alongside an interpreter** **Parental report: Language case history, plus *consider* direct assessment** | |
| --- | --- | --- |
| | Verbal comprehension | Expressive language |
| Early years | Parental report, such as the MacArthur-Bates CDI in home language. Informal assessment using culturally appropriate play with real objects and toys. Informal assessment using wordless books and culturally adapted or culturally appropriate pictures. Observation of interactions with other children from the same language community. | |
| 3;6–6;0 | Optional assessment of verbal comprehension skills using a culturally and linguistically adapted informal assessment | Assess expressive language skills in home language – basic sentences and early concepts |
| 6:0+ | Optional assessment of verbal comprehension skills using a culturally and linguistically adapted informal assessment | Assess expressive language including sequencing and narrative via storytelling. Wordless, culturally appropriate picture materials may be needed especially if the language is preliterate. |

**Key considerations:**
Check that names of any objects used in assessment.
Does the family use a home language word, a borrowing or codeswitch?
Does the child perceive the setting to be an additional language setting (this pragmatic pressure is especially strong in educational settings)?
Do not assume that language will be developed from simple to complex *in one language*. The child or young person may have the concept or vocabulary in their other language(s).
Children may acquire "later"/"'harder" and seemingly more complex sentence structures and concepts before "easier" ones. For example, prepositions before simple sentences.

**Comorbidity**
Does the child have:
• Poor vocabulary
• Speech Sound Disorder
• Dysfluency
• Other speech, language, or communication need?

## Diagnosis of SLCN, Language Difficulties, and Developmental Language Disorder

"Language delay" is no longer an acceptable diagnosis. This is because it implies the child will eventually catch up and this is often not the case. The diagnosis of "delayed language" or "language delay" is frequently applied to children growing up in deprivation, with the implication that this is less serious than other causes of Language Difficulties, despite no support for this view in the research literature (Bishop et al., 2016).

Bilingual children who are assessed in only the additional language may be labelled as "delayed" in that language. This is incorrect and fails to consider the child's whole language functioning. If the child has no difficulties in their home language, then they are a potential or emerging bilingual speaker. With sufficient exposure to the additional language, they will develop typical language skills in both/all languages they hear and speak.

Young children with language problems that "significantly impair social and/or educational functioning with indicators of poor prognosis" (Ebbels, 2020) should be diagnosed with "Speech, Language, and Communication Needs" (SLCN) or "Language Difficulties." Children under the age of 5 who still experience difficulties which meet the above description, or those under that age who are likely to continue experiencing difficulties until they are 5;0 and over, should be diagnosed with "Developmental Language Disorder" (DLD). Children may also have a biomedical condition, and this does not necessarily cause the language disorder. Please see Bishop et al. (2016); Norbury et al. (2016); Ebbels (2020) and Pert (2020) for a full overview of recent terminology.

None of this terminology would refer to bilingual children simply because they cannot speak the mainstream language. SLCN, Language Disorder, DLD or DLD associated with a biomedical condition would be recognised in a bilingual child as they would experience difficulties in both/all their languages.

### Codeswitching and the myth of word/phrase order errors

It was thought that children with language disorder made qualitative errors in their expressive language, specifically, the construction of spoken sentences or spoken utterances. A review of several different languages by Leonard concluded that "Children with SLI whose language permits considerable variation in word order will show greater word order variation than children with SLI acquiring a language with rigid word order" (1998, p. 117). Note that "Specific Language Impairment" (SLI) was the accepted terminology for

Developmental Language Disorder (DLD) at that time. Children look like poorer speakers of *their particular language.*

The myth of word/phrase order errors seems to persist for children exposed to a home language that contrasts with the language of education, in the guise of "interference." Children may be described as being "confused" by being exposed to more than one language and making errors because the home language is affecting their acquisition of the additional language.

Although there are undoubtedly influences of one language on another, especially in the very early stages of language acquisition, children rarely fail to comply with the language structure for the language they are using. In a study of children aged 3;0 to 7;5 living in the UK with a home language of Mirpuri, only three utterances from a total of 583 codeswitched utterances (0.52%) did not conform to the monolingual word/phrase order or morphological structure of Mirpuri (Pert, 2007). This shows that when two or more languages are involved in an utterance, one language sets the morphosyntactic frame, while content words may be drawn from any of the child's languages. This supports the matrix language and 4M models proposed by Myers-Scotton (2002).

Monolingual speakers may perceive children learning two or more languages to have a delay in acquiring each language. This perception comes from evaluating only one of the child's languages and that usually is the language of education (English). Bilingual child is not to monolingual is in one. Bilingual children use codeswitched utterances that are of a similar length and complexity to their monolingual peers. However, for this to be observed available child must be in conversation with another bilingual person. This is because pragmatics restrained children from using both/all their languages with a person who they perceive to be monolingual.

If a child has a language disorder that this will be evident in both/all language that they speak. The best way to evaluate this is to examine the child's language ability across both/all languages rather than individually.

## Planning therapy in home language: dynamic assessment

Dynamic assessment has long been used to evaluate bilingual children's language learning capabilities. This approach is descriptive and uses the child as their own baseline. This avoids the need to use standardised assessments, which are often misleading when

**Table 6.9** Bilingual language acquisition versus diagnosis of SLCN, Language Difficulties, or Developmental Language Disorder (DLD)

| Skills in the home language | Skills in the additional language | Comment | Diagnosis |
|---|---|---|---|
| Typical home language skills | Not yet developed | Potential bilingual: No exposure/minimal exposure to additional language | **Not applicable:** Sequential bilingual child typically aged 1;0 to 3;6 years depending on first exposure to the additional language |
| Typical home language skills | Emerging additional language skills (Not at the level of monolingual peers) | Sequential bilingual: Start of the process of additional language learning <2 years exposure to additional language | **Not applicable:** Sequential bilingual child typically aged 3;6 to 6;0 years depending on first exposure to the additional language |
| Typical home language skills | Basic interpersonal conversational skills (BICS) | Sequential bilingual: 2+ years exposure to additional language | **Not applicable:** Sequential bilingual child typically aged 5;6 to 7;0 years depending on first exposure to the additional language |
| Typical home language skills | Cognitive academic language proficiency (CALP) - Able to learn in the additional language | Sequential bilingual: 5-7 years exposure to additional language | **Not applicable:** Sequential bilingual who can use both languages at a level similar to a monolingual speaker. Typically, a child or young person aged 8;0 to 11;0+ depending on first exposure to the additional language |
| Poor home language skills | Not yet developed as not yet exposed to additional language | Child has not "cracked the code" for the only language they are exposed to | SLCN or Language Difficulties Typically, a child aged 1;0-3;6 years |
| Poor home language skills | Only just commenced additional language learning and exposure to additional language <2 years | Child has not "cracked the code" for any language | SLCN or Language Difficulties, or DLD if the child is likely to have problems that persist. Typically, a child aged 3;6-6;0 years depending on first exposure to the additional language |
| Poor home language skills | Poor additional language skills despite some time in an additional language setting 2+ years | Child has not "cracked the code" for any language | Developmental Language Disorder (DLD) Typically, a child aged 5;6 to 7;0 depending on first exposure to the additional language |

| Skills in the home language | Skills in the additional language | Comment | Diagnosis |
| --- | --- | --- | --- |
| Poor home language skills | Poor additional language skills despite some time in an additional language setting 5–7 years | Child has only partially "cracked the code" and has difficulty understanding and using *any language*. | Developmental Language Disorder (DLD) Typically, a child or young person aged 8:0–11+ years or above depending on first exposure to the additional language |

(*BICS* and *CALPS* adapted from Cummins, 2017)

**Table notes**

Developmental Language Disorder diagnosed after the age of 5 or before if problems are likely to persist past the age of 5. For young children where there are only very few indicators of poor prognosis use "Language Difficulties" or "Speech, Language, and Communication Needs" (SLCN) but NOT "Language Delay" or "Delayed Language."

Children with recognised aetiology may have a diagnosis of "Language Disorder Associated with X," where X is a biomedical condition such as a genetic condition, acquired brain injury, sensorineural hearing loss, intellectual disability, or autistic spectrum condition. (See Ebbels, 2020).

For a simultaneous bilingual child, "home language" is both/all the languages the child hears and uses. Comparison of other typically developing simultaneous bilingual children and/or estimates of exposure to each language should be made. It is not possible to apply normative data to the acquisition of two or more languages at home as the exposure from each carer will differ with each individual family.

translated unless properly culturally and linguistically adapted. Dynamic assessment is based on Vygotsky's model of cognitive development during social interactions with more capable adults (in this case the SLT). This leads to the child improving their skills in a shift from supported learning to independent skill (Gutiérrez-Clellen & Peña, 2001).

SLTs are familiar with supporting skills in young children. In the case of Dynamic Assessment, the assessment aims to identify *the amount of change the child can make when supported by the therapist*. If the child is only able to say two words in an utterance but can produce a three-word utterance when prompted with a sign or symbol, then we have discovered the "zone of proximal development" (ZPD).

The use of Dynamic Assessment focuses on the rate of development. Typically developing children will be able to move from adult-supported success to independent success within an episode of care. Whereas those children with Developmental Language Disorder will experience little or no success over the same time period and will require more input to achieve the same gains.

It is important to note here that an episode of care that is too short to allow the child to develop skills adequately may also lead to poor outcomes. Recall that when working with bilingual children, approximately double the time is required. Interventions for monolingual children require sufficient dosage or treatment intensity to be effective. An episode of care lasting fewer than eight weeks is likely to be less effective than intervention lasting eight weeks or more (Law et al., 2003). Interventions delivered more than once a week more effective than once weekly input, even if the same overall contact time is the same across the episode of care (Allen, 2013). The traditional six-week block often encountered in the UK is not evidence-based and should be robustly challenged. For bilingual children, an episode of sixteen weeks or more, with two-three sessions per week is likely to be required to effect significant progress.

Although the Dynamic Assessment approach has been proposed as a way of working in the mainstream language when home language interpreters are not available, this is strongly discouraged. Working exclusively in the mainstream language gives the message that home language is not relevant and reinforces the incorrect message that the mainstream language (usually English) is the only important language for educational success.

It is recommended that a Dynamic Assessment approach in the mainstream language is only adopted after all efforts have been made to secure an interpreter in the home language. Barriers such as funding and costs should *never* be used as an excuse for not working alongside an interpreter (Royal College of Speech and Language Therapists, 2021).

Dynamic assessment is now also recommended for the assessment of children with Developmental Language Disorder (DLD) (Hasson & Botting, 2010; Hasson et al., 2012).

Language domains which have been investigated using Dynamic Assessment include:

- Narrative/Discourse
- Sentence level
- Semantics/word level/vocabulary
- Morphology
- Phonology

(Hasson, 2018; Orellana et al., 2019)

Many therapists will be familiar with the use of prompts in helping children to produce expressive language responses. The Dynamic Assessment approach takes this further, assessing the *type* and *level* of cues employed. The total number of cues can then be used as a baseline. The descriptive information on how the child was able to succeed with sufficient scaffolding is then used to plan intervention which is bespoke to that child's particular language needs (Hasson, 2018; Hasson et al., 2012).

This contrasts with a "model and repeat" approach, which is often employed in speech and language therapy sessions. This approach has several drawbacks, including the loss of interest in the shared attention activity and likely bypassing of the semantic system. Asking people learning foreign vocabulary to imitate spoken words in order to learn new vocabulary has been shown to be less effective than asking them to try and name the item and then receive feedback (Kang et al., 2013). Note that this is not the same as learning being enhanced by hearing words and phrases repeatedly in the language *input*, but rather about how we go about asking children to *use* language.

Similarly, using simplified utterances (telegraphic utterances such as "man eat apple" instead of "*the* man *is* eat*ing an* apple") is not recommended (Fey et al., 2003), as this reduces the number of cues a child has. For example, a determiner in English helps predict that a noun is next. A gender agreement morpheme in Punjabi helps to identify ACTIONS in utterances.

In order to deliver a Dynamic Assessment session in home language, careful planning is required for the task(s) to be presented. A planning session with the interpreter will ensure that any questions about the prompts to be provided are answered before meeting the child or young person.

Consider the prompt sheet for the *Dynamic Assessment of Sentence Structure* (DASS) (Hasson et al., 2012). The words underlined would likely need some discussion on exactly how they are translated and presented to the child or young person. The interpreter might also be unfamiliar with cloze: missing off the final word for the child to supply, such as "The man is eating an . . . ." Concepts such as "swop" and "different" (in relation to words) may also be culturally and linguistically different in a particular language.

For a session on spoken sentences using this approach, the interpreter and SLT would need to list a set of cues in the home language transliterated by the therapist. The therapist could then follow the session, recognising the home-language cues provided. The debrief session would then discuss the child's performance and check the expressive language and any cues provided by the interpreter. In this way, use of (mainly) home-language and/or code-switched responses would be encouraged.

**Table 6.10** Dynamic assessment cue levels

| Cue level | Description of cue | Example of phrasing | Home language cue transliterated |
|---|---|---|---|
| 1. | Metacognitive direction spontaneous response | Do you know what you have to do? | |
| 2. | Drawing on previous knowledge | How did you do this <u>before</u>?<br>Do you know all the words?<br>Is that right? Can you <u>fix</u> it? | |
| 3. | Finding strategies | Which one can you <u>start</u> with?<br>You need to start with <u>something different</u> this time<br>Can you make <u>little groups of words</u>?<br>Can you make a question?<br>Can you <u>swop</u> the words around? | |
| | Problem solving | Have you used all the words?<br>What have you left out?<br>Reminder - "Last time you said" | |
| 4. | Breaking down the task | Which one shall we start with?<br>Which one can you start with to make a question?<br>Start with . . . X.<br>What comes <u>next</u>? | |
| | Using specific feedback | You have <u>left this one out</u> - where does it go?<br><u>Repeat</u> part of answer already used<br>Giving part of answer | |
| 5. | Learning from feedback and instruction | Scaffolding sentence bit by bit<br>Presenting <u>cloze task</u><br>Explaining.<br>Identifying errors<br>Modelling for imitation | |
| | Reflection - when the answer is correct | Is that the right answer?<br>Why was it not ok?<br>Can you tell me how you did that?<br>How did you know how to do that?<br>Was it easy or hard? Why? | |

(Adapted from Hasson et al., 2012, p. 290)

## Delivering therapy in home language

RCSLT clinical guidelines are clear that assessment and therapy should be in the child's home language for the best outcomes (Royal College of Speech and Language Therapists, 2021). The aim of all intervention with bilingual children is to maintain and develop home language skills to the best of the child's ability. This is a similar approach to therapy with monolingual children. That is, to help the child to maximise their communication skills. Despite this clear clinical guidance, the experience of bilingual families is that they are often only offered assessment and therapy in English.

## Therapy aims: examples

A Care Plan should be written setting out the episode of care therapy aims, resources required and the language(s) in which the intervention will be delivered. This Care Plan may then be shared with the parent(s)/carer and other interested professionals in the multidisciplinary team, such as teaching staff.

The Care Plan should be shared with parent(s)/carer as a written document (so that family can show the plan to others), AND as a verbal version. This may be achieved by asking the parent(s)/carer to video the interpreter and therapist explaining the programme in home language. This may then be shared with others not present at the appointment, such as the extended family who may be keen to assist in the delivery of the planned therapy in home language.

Notes:
- Therapy aims/goals/targets should be measurable and refer to a change in the child or young person's language which can be observed (comprehension) or heard (expression).
- Aims worded as "To attempt to . . ." or "To try to . . ." mean that the aims are completed as soon as the episode of care commences and so should be avoided.
- Aims such as "To be able to . . ." are verbose and can as easily be expressed as "To . . ."
- Aims which involve assessment or tasks for the therapist or adults are not aims as they do not involve a change in the child's abilities. Examples include "To assess X's expressive language." These are a "to-do" list for the therapist and should be included in diaries and planning documents, not in Care Plans.

For young children with language disorder, using full spoken utterances may be a key therapy aim. The following are possible therapy aims for the *Building Early Sentences Therapy* programme (Adapted from McKean et al., 2013b) organised by language level.

## Examples of therapy aims for basic spoken utterances in Mirpuri

The comments illustrate difference that need to be considered when translating therapy aims. The aims cannot be directly translated. Unsurprisingly, languages have different ways of encoding meaning. Other languages will of course have different aspects to consider.

Providing home language therapy aims gives real examples for the parent(s)/carer to consider, since most parents will not have training in linguistics. Moreover, pre-planning these therapy aims with the interpreter will enable the clinician to recognise any adaptations to their approach and select culturally appropriate therapy materials. The parent(s)/carer will also have more trust that the clinician understands their child's needs if they can discuss actual examples of home language words or utterances and highlight how the child's responses differ from the targets, despite not being able to speak the family's home language fluently.

## Syntactic targets

These targets are for children who cannot combine words into spoken utterances.

- To produce a range of spoken utterances including an **AGENT** and **ACTION**,
  For example,
  - / **qɑqɑ tuɾ**-na pi-ja /
  *baby walk-ing + male is + male*
  (The) **baby** (he) is **walking**
- To produce a range of spoken utterances including an **AGENT, ACTION** and **PATIENT**,
  For example,
  - / **kʊɾi kɑp** qi **qɪq mɑɾ**-ni pi/
  *girl cup to kick doing + contact + female is + female*
  (The) **girl** (she) is **kick**ing (a) **cup**

## Vocabulary targets

These are for children who have not yet acquired a range of nominal vocabulary

- To use a range of (6) **AGENTS**,
  - / d͡ʒəna/(*man*),
  - / d͡ʒənani/(*woman/lady*),
  - / kʊɾi/(*girl*),
  - / mʊɾa/(*boy*),
  - / qɑqɑ/(*baby*),
  - "**teddy**" (English borrowing) (*teddy (bear)*).

To use a range of (24) **PATIENTS**, including:

- / **seːb**/(*apple, masculine*);
- / **mɑlʈɑ**/(*orange, masculine*);
- / **keːlɑ**/(*banana, masculine*);
- / **gad͡ʒəɾ** / (*carrot*);

- **lolly(pop)** *(English borrowing)*
- / t͡ʃʌmʌt͡ʃ/*(spoon)*;
- / kæ̃p/*(cup, English borrowing)*;
- / bɪli/*(cat, female)*;
- **cycle** *(bike/bicycle, English borrowing)*;
- / pʰʊl/*(flower)*;
- / d͡ʒurɑb/*(sock)*;
- / gḛ̃ɳɖ / *(ball)*;
- / d͡ʒuʈ i/*(shoes)*;
- / bərʌʃ / t͡ʃɑɽu/*(brush, English borrowing/home language word)*;
- / d͡ʒabi/*(key)*;
- **Phone** *((tele)phone, English borrowing)*;
- / mẽz/*(table)*;
- / ɓɪstɽ / *(bed)*;
- / ɖ ʊɖ / *(milk)*;
- / dʌba/*(box)*;
- / maltẽna d͡ʒus/or/maltẽna ɾæs/*(oranges of juice; juice)*.
- **Note that in Mirpuri, nouns have gender** (masculine, feminine; or plural form).
- **The gender of the noun also interacts with some adjectives.**

*Grammatical targets*

### Action (verb) targets

These targets are for children who have not yet acquired a range of verbs.

- To produce (two) **intransitive verbs** (AGENT + ACTION),
  - / **beh**-ta va/or/**beh**-ti vi' /

    *sit-ing + male is + male or sit-ing + female is + female*
  - / **tuɾ**-na pija/or/**tuɾ**-ni pi /

    *walk-ing + male is + male or walk-ing + female is + female*
- To produce a range of (four) **transitive verbs**
- **Mirpuri has an AGENT + PATIENT + ACTION phrase structure**
  - / mʌɽa gʊɖi ki ʈ õ-ɳa pi-ja /

    *boy doll to wash-ing + male is + male*

    *(The) boy (he) is washing (a) doll*
  - / mʌɽa pʰʊɫ sʌŋgə-ɳa pi-ja /

    *boy flowers smell-ing + male is + male*

    *(The) boy (he) is smelling (some) flowers*
  - d͡ʒənani bərʌʃ / t͡ʃɑɽu maɾ-ni pi

lady/woman brush do + contact-ing + female is + female

(The) lady is brushing

- Mirpuri verbs have one auxiliary verb form for intransitive verbs (va/vi) and another for monotransitive and ditransitive verbs (pi-ja/pi).
- Mirpuri has a verb structure where a noun + dummy do verb form is used (see "brushing," above). This includes "mar" (where one item contacts another, such as "brushing" or "hitting") and "kar" (Pert, 2007).
- Mirpuri present progressive agrees with the gender of the AGENT.

**Phrase level targets – noun phrases and verb phrases**

These targets are for children who only use a single word or uninflected lexical item in a phrase.

- This therapy aim cannot be achieved in Mirpuri, as determiners are not part of the surface grammar of the language.
- To use an **auxiliary verb** *"is,"* e.g., "The man **is** eating an apple."
    - This therapy aim has two forms in Mirpuri. Mirpuri auxiliaries take the gender of the AGENT ("doer") of the ACTION. This is encoded as an /i/ vowel for female gender and /a/ for male gender:
        - / d͡ʒəna su-ʈa va /

        man sleep-ing + male is + male

        (The) man (he) is sleeping
        - / d͡ʒənani su-ʈi vi /

        lady/woman sleep-ing + female is + female

        (The) lady/woman (she) is sleeping

# When to introduce English (or Welsh or Gaelic)

Bilingual children living in the UK will inevitably need to use the language of the wider community. These are the languages of everyday life, education and of their peers.

This section will guide you on:

- When to introduce additional language targets
- How to advise education staff on the use of the majority language
- Handling attitudes to codeswitching (using two languages together in the same conversation or even the same spoken sentence)

## Monitoring progress

Assessing the timing of therapy and the progress a child makes is challenging for the SLT to judge for any client. For bilingual children, this is especially difficult, as many families may have difficulty recording home practice, and may need additional support to implement therapy programmes at home.

The use of technology such as video recording, video calls and lo-tech strategies such as observing the family carry out practice in clinic and providing feedback alongside an interpreter should be explored.

## The impact of teachers' attitude to home languages

Teachers often believe that children should speak the mainstream language. Bezcioglu-Göktolga and Yagmur (2018) found that Dutch speaking teachers working with Turkish-Dutch bilingual children "advise parents that they should speak Dutch to their children as soon as children start school. Accordingly, if children need to make a preference, this should always be Dutch" (230).

Teachers often feel unprepared for dealing with multilingual pupils, leading to a banning of home language in the classroom, due to the belief that all the available time should be dedicated to learning the mainstream language (Van Der Wildt et al., 2017).

Even when teachers are positive about bilingualism, educational leaders place responsibility for language maintenance or attrition and loss on parents and children, rather than taking personal or institutional responsibility to enhance home language use in school (Cunningham, 2020).

Formal use of home language, although encouraged in the UK, is seldom if ever implemented in reality. Bailey and Marsden (2017, p. 297) reported that in 15 hours of observation "children's home languages were not evidenced either visually or interactionally, and no instances of any languages other than English being used were observed."

SLTs therefore have a role in training teachers about bilingualism, but also helping to implement home language usage both for therapy programmes, but also more widely in the policy of language choice in the classroom. Children benefit both educationally and from a socio-emotional perspective when they experience affirmation of their home language(s) in the classroom. Limiting this to "show and tell" and other peripheral activities is unlikely to maintain their home language skills.

**Table 6.11** Comparison of language assessments and interventions

| ASSESSMENT/ INTERVENTION TYPE | MEASURE(S) | ADVANTAGES | DRAWBACKS |
|---|---|---|---|
| **Static/snapshot assessment** | | | |
| Informal assessment of expressive language in home language(s) using toys, objects and pictures/ photographs reflecting the child or young person's culture. | Mean Length of Utterance (MLU). MLU words may be as useful as MLU morphemes (Parker & Brorson, 2005). Descriptive analysis of errors, omissions and lack of/ disordered codeswitching. | Culturally and linguistically appropriate. Best possible language sample. Can be analysed on computer for faster and more accurate results (See Pezold et al., 2020). | No normative data OR use stages and developmental data from published research on home language/bilingual acquisition where available. Language sampling and MLU calculations can be time-consuming unless familiar with using a template and computerised analysis (training recommended). |
| Informal assessment of verbal comprehension of home language(s) using toys, objects and pictures/ photographs reflecting the child or young person's culture. | Complexity of instructions. | Provides an idea of ability to follow instructions. | Cannot use Information Carry Words (ICWs) reliably as, unlike English, most languages have more than one piece of information mapped onto different morphemes and/or syntactic structures |
| Adapted published standardised assessment, such as the New Reynell Developmental Language Scales using the Multilingual Toolkit delivered in home language(s) | Raw Scores. Descriptive information. | Culturally and linguistically adapted. | Cannot quote normative data (age equivalents; percentile ranks; standard scores) as these relate only to monolingual English children (unless re-standardised on other populations) |
| Published standardised assessment translated into home language(s) but not adapted | Raw Scores. Descriptive information. | Child may fail items due to cultural issues. Child may not recognise activities, objects, people, or settings Some items will not translate to the same surface structures – differences in complexity. Some concepts/items will not exist in home language. | Misleading information provided as the test is not fit for the purpose of assessing bilingual children. Inherently discriminatory and highly likely to disadvantage home language children and young people, and those from different cultures. Strongly advise not to select this option. |

| ASSESSMENT/ INTERVENTION TYPE | MEASURE(S) | ADVANTAGES | DRAWBACKS |
|---|---|---|---|
| Published standardised assessment delivered in English (or other mainstream language) | Descriptive information. | Child likely to be disadvantaged by cultural and linguistic differences to their own lived experience. Assessment of only one language ignores skills in home language(s) leading to inappropriate/ incorrect diagnosis. Invalid approach, viewing the bilingual child as two monolingual speakers in one. | Use of age equivalents, standard scores, percentile ranks, or other scores compare the child unfairly with monolingual peers. High risk of completely invalid conclusions. This option should never be selected as it is inherently discriminatory. |
| **Parental report** | | | |
| Parental report of vocabulary knowledge and naming. Parental report of best/ longest utterances. | Categories of words Number of referents, or total conceptual vocabulary (Swain, 1972 in De Houwer et al., 2014). | Can apply across both/all languages (referents rather than both labels in two languages, for example). | Some families will be accurate reporting, while different caring arrangements may make this more challenging for other families. For example, a grandparent and older sibling may take the lead on caring for a young child. Tends to be practical for young children only. |
| **Dynamic assessment** | | | |
| Dynamic assessment in home language | Zone of proximal development. Number and level of cues provided. | Bespoke therapy aims for the child or young person. Avoid use of static assessments. Culturally and linguistically valid. | Not able to compare children easily. |
| Dynamic assessment in mainstream language such as English | Zone of proximal development. Number and level of cues provided. | Bespoke therapy aims for the child or young person. Avoid use of static assessments. May be culturally valid. | Reinforces the view that the mainstream language is more important than home language. Intervention in the mainstream language likely to speed-up home language attrition. Failure to involve adult to inform about cultural barriers increases likelihood of failure to achieve targets. |

*(Continued)*

**Table 6.11** (Continued)

| ASSESSMENT/ INTERVENTION TYPE | MEASURE(S) | ADVANTAGES | DRAWBACKS |
|---|---|---|---|
| **Intervention** | | | |
| Home language programme set using bespoke therapy aims/targets/goals based on descriptive assessment | MLU (words) or MLU (morphemes). Achievement of set therapy aims. Translated/adapted WHO ICF based outcome measure, such as the FOCUS (Thomas-Stonell et al., 2013) | Culturally and linguistically meets the needs of the child or young person and their family. Family able to practice at home. Develops/maintains home language and enhances sense of identity and wellbeing. Best possible outcomes. | *Perceived* drawbacks are financial, and include: <br> • Working alongside an interpreter <br> • At least double the time compared to working with a family with whom you share a language <br> Commissioners and team leads should know that the requirements to work in this way are **not optional** and that financial constraints are not a valid reason to deny funding for the care pathway. |
| Intervention using a published programme in the mainstream language | Programme specific. | None. Expedient for professionals at the cost of appropriate outcomes for the client and their family. Embeds organisational racism. | Not culturally or linguistically sensitive. Encourages home language attrition. Risk to sense of identity and relationships with parent(s) and extended family. Risk to engagement with home language-speaking community in the future and opportunities to participate in culture. |

**Notes**

Total conceptual vocabulary (TCV) in bilingual children counts the number of concepts or lexical meanings. Therefore, if a bilingual child knows the word in both their languages, this forms a translation equivalent pair. In a Mirpuri speaking child who knows both "topi" and "hat," they have a TE **pair** relating to **one** lexical item or referent. Using this approach, De Houwer et al. (2014) stated that "our study finds no evidence of consistent differences between young bilinguals' and monolinguals' vocabulary sizes," although this study examined simultaneous Dutch-French bilingual families and not sequential bilingual families.

# References

Allen, M. M. (2013). Intervention efficacy and intensity for children with speech sound disorder. *Journal of Speech, Language, and Hearing Research, 56*, 865–877. https://doi.org/10.1044/1092-4388(2012/11-0076)

Ambridge, B., & Lieven, E. V. M. (2011). *Child language acquisition contrasting theoretical approaches.* Cambridge University Press.

Avramidis, E., & Koehn, P. (2008). *Enriching morphologically poor languages for statistical machine translation. ACL-08: HLT* (pp. 763–770). Association for Computational Linguistics. https://www.aclanthology.org/P08-1087.pdf

Bailey, E. G., & Marsden, E. (2017). Teachers' views on recognising and using home languages in predominantly monolingual primary schools. *Language and Education, 31*, 283–306. https://doi.org/10.1080/09500782.2017.1295981

Bezcioglu-Göktolga, I., & Yagmur, K. (2018). The impact of Dutch teachers on family language policy of Turkish immigrant parents. *Language, Culture, and Curriculum, 31*, 220–234. https://doi.org/10.1080/07908318.2018.1504392

Bishop, D. V. M., Snowling, M. J., Thompson, P. A., Greenhalgh, T., & Consortium, C. (2016). CATALISE: A multinational and multidisciplinary Delphi consensus study. Identifying language impairments in children. *PLoS One, 11*(7), e0158753. https://doi.org/10.1371/journal.pone.0158753

Broomfield, J., & Dodd, B. (2004). Children with speech and language disability: Caseload characteristics. *International Journal of Language & Communication Disorders, 39*(3), 303–324. https://doi.org/10.1080/13682820310001625589

Cummins, J. (2017). BICS and CALP: Empirical and theoretical status of the distinction. In *Cham: Springer international publishing* (pp. 59–71). https://doi.org/10.1007/978-3-319-02252-9_6

Cunningham, C. (2020). When 'home languages' become 'holiday languages': Teachers' discourses about responsibility for maintaining languages beyond English. *Language, Culture, and Curriculum, 33*, 213–227. https://doi.org/10.1080/07908318.2019.1619751

Dale, P. (2015). *MacArthur-bates CDI: Adaptations, not translations.* CDI Advisory Board. https://www.mb-cdi.stanford.edu/documents/AdaptationsNotTranslations2015.pdf

De Houwer, A., Bornstein, M. H., & Putnick, D. L. (2014). A bilingual-monolingual comparison of young children's vocabulary size: Evidence from comprehension and production. *Applied Psycholinguistics, 35*, 1189–1211. https://doi.org/10.1017/S0142716412000744

Eadie, P., Morgan, A., Ukoumunne, O. C., Ttofari Eecen, K., Wake, M., & Reilly, S. (2015). Speech sound disorder at four years: Prevalence, comorbidities, and predictors in a community cohort of children. *Developmental Medicine & Child Neurology, 57*(6), 578–584. https://doi.org/10.1111/dmcn.12635

Ebbels, S. (2020, November 4). *Webinar: DLD – When is a diagnosis appropriate?* Wednesday. Royal College of Speech and Language Therapists. Retrieved July 27, 2021, from http://www.rcslt.org/events/dld-when-is-a-diagnosis-appropriate

Fey, M. E., Long, S. H., & Finestack, L. H. (2003). Ten principles of grammar facilitation for children with specific language impairments. *American Journal of Speech Language Pathology, 12*, 3–15. https://doi.org/10.1044/1058-0360(2003/048).

Griffiths, C. (2008). Colonial education. In P. Poddar, R. S. Patke, L. Jensen, J. Beverley, C. Forsdick, P.-P. Fraiture, P. P., R. Ben-Ghiat, T. Dh'aen, B. Kundrus, E. Monasterios, & P. Rothwell (Eds.), *A historical companion to postcolonial literatures – Continental Europe and its empires* (pp. 124–125). Edinburgh University Press. www.jstor.org/stable/10.3366/j.ctt1g0b6vw.62

Gutiérrez-Clellen, V. F., & Peña, E. (2001). Dynamic assessment of diverse children: A tutorial. *Language, Speech and Hearing Services in Schools, 32*(4), 212–224.

Hasson, N. (2018). *The dynamic assessment of language learning.* Routledge. https://doi.org/10.4324/9781315175423

Hasson, N., & Botting, N. (2010). Dynamic assessment of children with language impairments: A pilot study. *Child Language Teaching and Therapy, 26*, 249–272. https://doi.org/10.1177/0265659009349982

Hasson, N., Dodd, B., & Botting, N. (2012). Dynamic Assessment of Sentence Structure (DASS): Design and evaluation of a novel procedure for the assessment of syntax in children with language impairments. *International Journal of Language & Communication Disorders, 47*, 285–299. https://doi.org/10.1111/j.1460-6984.2011.00108.x

Hendriks, P., & Spenader, J. (2005). When production precedes comprehension: An optimization approach to the acquisition of pronouns. *Language Acquisition, 13*(4), 319–348. https://doi.org/10.1207/s15327817la1304_3

Kang, S. H. K., Gollan, T. H., & Pashler, H. (2013). Don't just repeat after me: Retrieval practice is better than imitation for foreign vocabulary learning. *Psychonomic Bulletin & Review, 20*, 1259-1265. https://doi.org/10.3758/s13423-013-0450-z

Law, J., Garrett, Z., & Nye, C. (2003). Speech and language therapy interventions for children with primary speech and language delay or disorder. *The Cochrane Database of Systematic Reviews*, Article No: CD004110. https://doi.org/10.1002/14651858.CD004110

Leonard, L. B. (1998). *Children with specific language impairment*. MIT Press.

Letts, C., Edwards, S., Schaefer, B., & Sinka, I. (2014). The new reynell developmental language scales: Descriptive account and illustrative case study. *Child Language Teaching and Therapy, 30*, 103-116. https://doi.org/10.1177/0265659013492784

LIVELY: Language Intervention in the Early Years. (in press). *Polish and Sylheti adaptations of the new reynell developmental language scales using the multilingual toolkit*. https://www.research.ncl.ac.uk/lively/aboutlively.

McKean, C., Pert, S., & Stow, C. (2013a). *Building early sentences therapy: BEST manual*. Newcastle University and Pennine Care NHS Foundation Trust. https://www.research.ncl.ac.uk/media/sites/researchwebsites/languageinterventionintheearlyyears/BEST_Manual.pdf

McKean, C., Pert, S., & Stow, C. (2013b). *Building early sentences therapy: Aims for children*. Newcastle University and Pennine Care NHS Foundation Trust. www.buildingearlysentencestherapy.co.uk/resources/BEST-Care-plan-treatment-aims.pdf

Millar-Wilson, F. (2014, September 17). *FLAC: Functional language across countries: Development of resources for speech-language assessment in bilingualism*. Royal College of Speech and Language Therapists Conference: Mind the Gap: Putting Research into Practice.

Myers-Scotton, C. (2002). *Contact linguistics: Bilingual encounters and grammatical outcomes*. Oxford University Press. https://doi.org/10.1093/acprof:oso/9780198299530.001.0001.

Norbury, C. F., Gooch, D., Wray, C., Baird, G., Charman, T., Simonoff, E., . . . Pickles, A. (2016). The impact of nonverbal ability on prevalence and clinical presentation of language disorder: Evidence from a population study. *Journal of Child Psychology and Psychiatry, 57*, 1247-1257. https://doi.org/10.1111/jcpp.12573

Orellana, C. I., Wada, R., & Gillam, R. B. (2019). The use of dynamic assessment for the diagnosis of language disorders in bilingual children: A meta-analysis. *American Journal of Speech-Language Pathology, 28*, 1298-1317. https://doi.org/10.1044/2019_AJSLP-18-0202

Parker, M. D., & Brorson, K. (2005). A comparative study between mean length of utterance in morphemes (MLUm) and mean length of utterance in words (MLUw). *First Language, 25*, 365-376. https://doi.org/10.1177%2F0142723705059114

Pert, S. (2007). *Bilingual language development in Pakistani heritage children in Rochdale UK: Intra-sentential codeswitching and the implications for identifying specific language impairment*. Unpublished PhD Thesis. Newcastle University. http://www.theses.ncl.ac.uk/jspui/handle/10443/2230.

Pert, S. (2020). DLD – When is a diagnosis appropriate? DLD in a bilingual context. In *DLD – When is a diagnosis appropriate?* Royal College of Speech and Language Therapists. http://www.youtube.com/watch?v=8uMOgNQCZrM

Pert, S., & Stow, C. (2003). *A translation protocol for speech and language therapists*. Paper presented at the 5th CPLOL Conference. www.research.manchester.ac.uk/portal/en/publications/a-traceable-translation-protocol-for-speech-and-language-therapy-teams-working-with-bilingual-clients(89991c4f-9f91-4da5-90db-c9fa8e1ef5cf).html

Pezold, M. J., Imgrund, C. M., & Storkel, H. L. (2020). Using computer programs for language sample analysis. *Language, Speech & Hearing Services in Schools, 51*, 103-114. https://doi.org/10.1044/2019_LSHSS-18-0148

Rowland, M., Coombs, T., & Connor, M. (2019). A study of traveller horse owners' attitudes to horse care and welfare using an equine body condition scoring system. *Animals (Basel), 9*(4), 162. https://doi.org/10.3390/ani9040162

Royal College of Speech and Language Therapists. (2021). *Bilingualism guidance*. www.rcslt.org/members/clinical-guidance/bilingualism

Saeed, J. I. (2003). *Semantics second edition*. Blackwell.

Shriberg, L. D., Tomblin, J. B., & McSweeny, J. L. (1999). Prevalence of speech delay in six-year-old children and comorbidity with language impairment. *Journal of Speech, Language, and Hearing Research, 42*(6), 1461. https://doi.org/10.1044/jslhr.4206.1461

Stow, C., Pert, S., & Khattab, G. (2012). Translation to practice: Sociolinguistic and cultural considerations when working with the Pakistani Heritage community in England, UK. In S. McLeod & B. A. Goldstein (Eds.), *Multilingual aspects of speech sound disorders in children* (pp. 24-27). Multilingual Matters.

Thomas-Stonell, N., Oddson, B., Robertson, B., & Rosenbaum, P. (2013). Validation of the focus on the outcomes of communication under six outcome measure. *Developmental Medicine and Child Neurology, 55*, 546–552. https://doi.org/10.1111/dmcn.12123

Tomasello, M. (2003). *Constructing a language: A usage-based theory of language acquisition.* Harvard University Press.

Van Der Wildt, A., Van Avermaet, P., & Van Houtte, M. (2017). Opening up towards children's languages: Enhancing teachers' tolerant practices towards multilingualism. *School Effectiveness and School Improvement, 28*, 136–152. https://doi.org/10.1080/09243453.2016.1252406

# SPEECH SOUND DISORDER IN A BILINGUAL CONTEXT

DOI: 10.4324/9781003125563-7

## Speech Sound Disorder

Speech Sound Disorder (SSD) is the most frequently encountered communication disorder affecting children. Almost one in three children referred for speech and language therapy in the UK have speech difficulties, estimated to be 6.4% of annual live births, or 29.1% of referrals (Broomfield & Dodd, 2004a). However, estimates vary widely due to different classification, definitions and criteria for the acquisition of speech sounds (Dodd et al., 2006).

Prevalence refers to the number of children living with Speech Sound Disorder at any given time. This changes with the age profile, the community or country and the definition of SSD employed. This means figures vary depending on the study. For example, Eadie et al. (2015) reported that 3.4% of children at 4 years of age had SSD (Australia). ASHA (2020) in the US reports 2.3% to 24.6% of school-aged children.

There is a high level of overlap, or co-morbidity with language disorder. Broomfield and Dodd (2004b) found that one-third of children with SSD also had expressive language disorder, and half had semantic difficulties.

As bilingualism never causes or contributes to a speech, language, or communication disorder, it is likely that children speaking two or more languages will experience SSD at a similar rate to their monolingual peers.

We do need to consider that SSD is associated with physical aspects (the vocal tract) and psycholinguistic aspects (phonology). Since phonology is the system that allows language to be encoded for transmission to a listener, it is the interface between abstract language and concrete speech (sound waves). Phonology relies on contrast to signal different meanings within a particular language. We can therefore expect to encounter different phonological systems, and speech sound errors caused by under specification of these contrasts. In other words, the type of phonological errors observed are likely to be language dependant.

## SSD and literacy

Poor phonological awareness skills lead to a higher risk of literacy difficulties, and children with SSD are likely to have poor phonological skills in comparison to their typically developing peers (Brosseau-Lapré & Roepke, 2019).

It is unclear if phonological awareness arises *as a result* of developing a full phonological system or if phonological awareness *drives* phonological development. Hesketh et al. (2000) found little difference between the outcomes for children with SSD receiving an articulation-based therapy and a metaphonological approach. Similarly, the children with SSD did not have significantly different outcomes if they had poor or good initial phonological awareness skills.

It is therefore advisable to include production work in all therapy sessions and not use an exclusively phonological awareness-based approach.

## Phonological awareness

Nursery rhymes are often an integral part of childhood and are culturally appropriate for English speaking children. However, this is not true for other languages, such as Urdu, where rhyme in the form of poetry is the domain of high-status adults. Rhyme is also not thought to evoke change in children's phonology, but rather assist children in recognising rhyme in literacy. The assumption that phonological awareness leads to better literacy has been challenged, especially for children living in deprivation by Nancollis et al. (2005, p. 332) who stated "intervention focusing on syllable and rhyme awareness does not boost literacy acquisition as hoped."

## Literacy and phonological awareness in a bilingual context

Many languages are pre-literate, that is, have no written form, or are in the early stages of developing a script. Highly literate SLTs will not have experience of what it is like to develop a language purely through aural and verbal means. We assume that all speakers organise their language in the same way. This is to underestimate the profound effect of literacy. For example, a bilingual speech and language therapy assistant was able to devise English word lists by initial phone in the same way as her monolingual English-speaking peers. However, when asked to do the same task in her home language, she was unable to consciously retrieve lexical items in this way. This is because her home language was pre-literate and so she had only retrieved words when they were required semantically and pragmatically. We had to sit together and go through the International Phonetic Alphabet and say possible word onsets to trigger word retrieval.

Languages do not have the same rules for the use and distribution of phonemes. Most people will be aware that languages other than English have phones that do not exist in

English. Just as importantly, it is important to recognise that the word positions phones may occur may also differ (phonotactic differences).

Consider the voiced velar nasal /ŋ/. In English phonology, it is only allowable word final and syllable final in words such as "ri**ng**"

/ ɹɪŋ/and/sɪŋ.ɪŋ /. It is never encountered word or syllable initial, and to do so would be considered disordered *[ŋəʊz].

In contrast, Mirpuri, a Pakistani-heritage language does allow the voiced velar nasal to occur word initial in words such as "grape" (ungur)/ŋːguɽ /.

## Suprasegmental phonology

The change in vocal pitch (frequency Hz) and loudness (intensity dB) may be used in speech to add additional information to the segments of speech (consonants and vowels). These aspects include:

- Tone – pitch across a word or syllable
- Primary word stress – relative prominence or loudness of one syllable compared to other syllables in the same multisyllabic word
- Intonation – maximum change in pitch on a tonic syllable or nucleus in an utterance

Other aspects to consider are that languages other than English may have different suprasegmental aspects including intonation, word stress, and tone (vocal pitch pattern).

Word stressor lexical stress is defined as "increased prominence placed on a certain syllable in a word" (Wayland, 2019, p. 52). Only multisyllabic words have a primary word stress, since monosyllabic words cannot have one syllable more prominent than another as there is only one syllable in the word. English word stress is a property of the lexical item. Changing the primary word stress can change the meaning of the word. Speakers of English as a foreign language may apply their own suprasegmental rules onto English words and stress a different syllable than a native speaker would. This may mark out an additional language speaker to a native speaker even if the segmental phonology (consonants and vowels) is on target.

English tends to have primary word stress on the first syllable for nouns, such as "dinosaur"/ˈdaɪ.nə.sɔ /, or "table"/ˈteɪ.bɬ / and/ˈslɪ.pə /. Suffixes and prefixes modify this rule. The IPA diacritic is a short vertical dash just prior to the primary stressed syllable.

Consider words that are similar in segmental form, such as "**pre**sent" (a gift) and "pre-**sent**" (to present or give to another person). The noun has the first syllable stressed, while the verb has the second syllable stressed. Similarly, "**re**cord" (vinyl disc) / "re**cord**" (to make a recording) and "**su**spect" (person suspected of a deed or crime) / "su**spect**" (the act of thinking someone has committed a deed or crime) have primary stress for the noun and stress on the second syllable for the action or verb. The picture for polysyllabic words is highly complex (see Wayland, 2019).

In addition to primary word stress, English speakers may also use intonation to highlight a particular word within a spoken utterance. Basic functions include:

- Making a statement using a *falling* vocal pitch
- Signalling a question by using a *rising* pitch
- Hesitation or uncertainty – *fall-rise* pitch pattern
- Exclamation, strong feeling – *rise-fall* pattern

(See Carr, 2013 for a full discussion of intonation patterns in English)

Note that the utterance intonation does not change the word primary stress.

For languages other than English, both word stress and intonation may function in very different ways. In addition, languages may also have a tonal contrast system where word meaning changes depending on the vocal pitch for that lexical item, even though the segmental phonology is identical.

For example, Lyallpuri Punjabi has a three-way tonal contrast:

Children with Speech Sound Disorder may fail to include these aspects or confuse them. Tonal disorders, like vowel disorders seem to be relatively rare and typically developing children acquire tones in the early years. So (2006) reported less than 1% of children made tone errors with children acquiring tonal contrasts by 2;0 years. Tonal contrasts seem to be established before segmental phonology (Li & Thompson, 1977; So, 2006).

**Table 7.1** Tonal system for Lyallpuri Punjabi

| MONOSYLLABIC WORDS | Lyallpuri Punjabi lexical item | English translation |
| --- | --- | --- |
| High | / t͡ʃá / | tea |
| Mid | / t͡ʃa / | enthusiasm |
| Low | / t͡ʃà / | peek |
| DISYLLABIC WORDS | | |
| High | / kə́ɽi/ | curry |
| Mid | / kəɽi / | a small bangle |
| Low | / kə̀ɽi / | watch |

(Adapted from Hussain et al., 2020, p. 294)

## Diagnostic labels and categories

**Speech Sound Disorder is not itself a diagnosis**, but rather a category of several different types of speech disorder. Depending on the model adopted, SSD may include motor speech difficulties with the physical production of sounds (articulation, oro-motor skills), the planning and execution of speech, and the encoding and sequencing of meaning into a contrastive speech code (phonology).

## Under-representation of bilingual children with SSD

In a comparison of monolingual English and Pakistani-heritage English bilingual children, Stow and Dodd (2005) highlighted that far fewer bilingual children were referred for SSD than their monolingual peers (25.74% bilingual children compared with 58.43%). The authors concluded that bilingual children with SSD were significantly under-represented, due to a combination of factors, including lack of home language screening assessments.

*Home language speech sound assessments*

Some authors have developed speech sound assessment tools in languages other than English. These include Stow & Pert's Bilingual Speech Sound Screen (BiSSS) (2020) for Mirpuri, Punjabi, and Urdu in a UK context. Construction of standardised screening tools requires more time than is generally available for routine clinical practice and should be undertaken as a formal research project.

In the absence of a published tool, informal assessments may be devised, but these will lack normative data and so exact diagnosis will not be possible.

## Low socioeconomic status as a risk factor for SSD

Low socioeconomic status is identified as one of the factors for increased risk of SSD (Wren, 2019). Not all bilingual children live in poverty. However, in the UK and in other parts of the world, many bilingual communities reside in areas of high socioeconomic deprivation. This factor alone has been shown to have negative effects on cognitive performance in adults (Naeem et al., 2018). Fernald et al. (2013, p. 244) found that "significant differences in both vocabulary learning and language processing efficiency that were already present by 18 months, with a 6-month gap emerging between higher- and lower-SES toddlers by 24 months." Vocabulary development is important for speech, since lexical and semantic knowledge links to the development of the phonological system.

## Discrimination based on ethnicity/language other than English use

Morgan et al. (2016, p. 195) found that in the US "Black children and Hispanic children from homes where a language other than English is spoken are less likely than otherwise similar white children to receive speech/language services." It is unclear if this difference in provision is linked to overt racism, to more subtle factors, such as uncertainty in how to work in languages other than English, or to lower expectations by professionals for Black and ethnic minority children.

## Causes of Speech Sound Disorder

For the majority of children presenting with SSD, there is no known cause or aetiology. Phonological Delay and phonological disorders are considered Speech Sound Disorders caused by psycholinguistic deficits that are not related to articulation or oromotor skills.

This is poorly understood by parents and many health professionals, who mainly look to physical causes for SSD, such as erroneous beliefs that tongue tie (whether present or not) prevents or delays speech development. A review by Webb et al. (2013, p. 645) concluded, "there is no strong evidence that ankyloglossia causes speech problems." Marshall et al. (2017) reported parents' negative views that bilingualism itself might cause speech and language disorders.

It is outside the remit of this book to review all the competing models of SSD, categorisation, and relative merits of any particular model. I will refer to Dodd's classification model since "Dodd's classification system is a potentially clinically useful classification tool"

(Waring & Knight, 2013, p. 33). The model is supported by a range of case studies, including those examining the model's application to bilingual children, and so is very relevant to this chapter.

## Separate phonological systems for each language

Dodd and her team demonstrated by a series of case studies that bilingual children develop separate phonological systems for each language they speak, with some interaction in the early years.

It is important to note that children have been observed to have the same underlying SSD, but that it is expressed in different ways in their languages. This includes:

- a phonological process observed in the speech of one language, but not another. For example, a child observed stopping /h/ in Mirpuri, "happy"/hʊʃ/➜ [kʊʃ], but not in English, "house" on target.
- Using the same phonological process in both languages but affecting different phonemes. For example, a child observed stopping /s/ to [t] in Mirpuri, but /f/ to [w] in English:
  - "clean"/sɑːf/ ➜ [tɑ];
  - "fishing"/ˈfɪ.ʃɪŋ/ ➜ [wɪtɪŋ] (Holm et al., 1999)

## One vocal tract – one articulatory system

Articulation is the **physical production** of phones using the vocal tract. It is very important to remember that articulation and phonology are not the same. **No one has ever heard or said a phoneme.** A person's phonological system is the way in which humans encode meaning into a speech code which can then be physically transmitted through the air. In speech, this is achieved by using the vocal tract to act on an airstream and realise phones (sounds). These sound waves are then propagated through the air to the listener.

The ear does the reverse; allowing sound waves to move the ear drum, and in turn the auditory ossicles which set up pressure waves in the cochlea. This activates hairs which in turn activate nerves. These signals are then interpreted as sound in the brain's auditory cortex.

This means that there are usually no gaps between words and the stream of phones means nothing to a person who speaks a different language. The encoding and the system of contrasts employed is unique to that particular language.

For most language speech is produced with egressive airstream (air coming up and out of the vocal tract via the mouth and nose). Some languages have non-pulmonic airstream mechanisms, including clicks.

A bilingual speaker will have two (or more), often very different encoding systems (phonologies), one phonological system for each language. The job of turning these contrasting coding systems into physical speech sounds is the role of the vocal tract. Any problem with single sound production will therefore affect both/all languages a child or young person speaks. This might include cleft lip and/or palate, but also missing teeth, malocclusion, or any physical difference that affects speech production.

## Classification of Speech Sound Disorder

**SSD is not a diagnosis**, but rather a heterogenous group of children. Dodd et al. (2005) classified monolingual English-speaking children with SSD into four subgroups. **These groups have also been observed in a range of languages other than English** and are regarded as robust categories for the classification of surface speech-errors (Holm et al., 1999, p. 275). Therefore, children with **suspected Speech Sound Disorder** have a confirmed diagnosis after assessment which replaces this more general category label (see Table 7.2).

Articulation impairment or articulation disorder

Articulation disorder is the inability to produce an acceptable and accurate realisation of a phoneme. The child produces a distortion or substitutes another phoneme. Articulation disorder is thought to be caused by a physical deficit in the vocal tract, such as missing teeth, open bite, and/or where an incorrect motor programme has been learnt.

It is important to differentiate an articulation disorder from a phonological disorder.

Children with an articulation disorder **will not be stimulable for a particular phoneme.** That is, they will not be able to imitate a sound in isolation, or in combination with vowels since they lack the physical ability to produce the sound.

### Articulation disorder: distortion

If the sound produced is not another phoneme of the language, then it will be classified as a **distortion.** In English monolingual children an example is when a voiceless alveolar fricative [s] is realised as a voiceless alveolar lateral fricative [ɬ] at sound and word level.

There is no change in meaning, since [ɬ] is not a phoneme of English and words where the phoneme /s/ is a segment are not confused with other lexical items.

Since phones in isolation have no meaning, they are transcribed in square brackets, such as [s]. In a stimulability assessment, each phone is therefore transcribed as:

[target phone] ➜ [realisation]

A child should be able to imitate an adult producing the single phone, providing that the child is old enough to have acquired that phone. If the child is old enough to have acquired that phone, and cannot imitate it accurately, then this is evidence of articulation disorder.

Articulation skills are the physical production of the phone in the vocal tract. Therefore, these may be assessed independently of language, that is, instructions may be provided in home language and the results will apply to any overlapping phones in English (or other languages spoken). However, consider that many languages will have phones not found in English, and that these should also be assessed.

Inventories of the phones of any particular language, and for some languages the age at which phonetic acquisition occurs have been researched and documented. It must be considered in which context the child you are assessing is acquiring their language(s), a monolingual or a bilingual/multilingual context. Normative data must be carefully matched so that the clinician only compares the child in question with the same population. Acquisition data for the monolingual context is likely to show earlier and/or different acquisition of phones and suppression of phonological processes than bilingual acquisition. See Hua and Dodd (2006) for further discussion and information on phonological inventories and ages of acquisition for several languages in a monolingual context including Putonghua (Modern Standard Chinese), Cantonese, Maltese, Telugu, Egyptian Arabic, and Turkish.

*Articulation disorder: articulation disorder with phonological implications*

If the sound **is another phoneme of the language**, then contrast in the phonological system cannot be signalled. This is **an articulation disorder with phonological implications**. This is easily confused with a phonological error, unless a stimulability assessment is undertaken. An example in English is when a voiceless alveolar fricative /s/ is realised as [t] at sound and word level. This might easily be mistaken for the phonological simplification process of "stopping," where a fricative is replaced by a plosive. However, the observation that the child is not able to physically produce the [s] realisation even as a single sound after an adult has provided a verbal model, demonstrates that this is a (physical/motor) articulation disorder and not a purely phonological disorder.

When a child **is stimulable**, that is, they **are** able to produce /s/ as [s] at sound level, but not in the context of meaningful words, then this would indicate a phonological difficulty, since the child has demonstrated no difficulty physically producing the sound (articulation disorder is not present).

It is important for both diagnosis and for planning intervention that articulation skills are examined outside the context of real words. For this reason, speech sound assessment should include a stimulability assessment for all sounds not realised on target in a word naming assessment. **Articulation Disorder may be present alongside a Phonological Delay or disorder.**

### Phonological Delay

Children with Phonological Delay have a similar system to that of a younger child. Most phonemes can be articulated (although articulation disorder may co-occur), but phonological simplification processes that most typically developing children have eliminated persist.

It is important to note that the presence of one or more unusual phonological process leads to a diagnosis of Consistent (atypical) Phonological Disorder, even if one or more phonological patterns consistent with delay are observed. Children with only delayed patterns are diagnosed with delayed phonological skills.

It is a common misconception that after a certain age, persisting Phonological Delay becomes phonological disorder. This is not the case. The therapist should refer to the simplification patterns observed in the child or young person's speech. I have encountered young people in their early 20s who have persisting Phonological Delay.

### Consistent (Atypical) Phonological Disorder

Unusual error patterns (with or without delayed processes) are indicative of Consistent Phonological Disorder. It is important to note that the child will typically have consistent lexical word production, that is <40% inconsistency. This can only be established by assessing at least 10 words twice on a confrontational single-word naming assessment.

## Inconsistent (or atypical) Phonological Disorder (IPD)

Variable production of the same word in the same context characterises Inconsistent Phonological Disorder. Motor sequencing planning is affected. Scores of > 40% inconsistency of **word production** are observed. It is important to note that inconsistency affects word production. It is not useful to state that a "phoneme is used inconsistently." Rather, the child may use separate rules for each word position. A detailed analysis which takes into account word positions and distribution is indicated.

**Table 7.2** Diagnoses

| Diagnosis 1 - Impairment at the Physical Level/Vocal Tract  LANGUAGE INDEPENDENT | | Diagnosis 2 - Impairment at the Psycholinguistic Level/Mapping meaning to a contrastive system  EACH LANGUAGE HAS A DIFFERENT SYSTEM |
|---|---|---|
| 1. | **None** Stimulable for all age-appropriate phones | **None** Phonological processes/error patterns observed in the child's speech are age-appropriate |
| 2. | **None** Stimulable for all age-appropriate phones | **Phonological Delay** Phonological simplification processes are observed in the child's speech which are found in younger children's speech |
| 3. | **None** Stimulable for all age-appropriate phones | **Consistent Phonological Disorder** Inconsistency of WORD production is <40% Phonological processes observed in the child's speech are NOT found in younger children's speech |
| 4. | **None** Stimulable for all age-appropriate phones | **Inconsistent Phonological Disorder** Inconsistency of WORD production is >40% No phonological process as words are realised differently on each attempt (no pattern) |
| 5. | **Articulation disorder** Distortions: Child is not stimulable/ cannot imitate phones that s/he should be able to at this age. Errors are not phonemes of either/any of the languages | **Same errors at word level as at sound level** NB. The errors are distortions and do not trigger a change in meaning |
| 6. | **Articulation disorder with phonological implications** Substitutions: Child is not stimulable/cannot imitate phones that s/he should be able to at this age. Errors result in another phoneme of one or more of the languages spoken | **Same errors at word level as at sound level** NB. The errors may *appear* to be phonological processes as the articulation errors result in substitution with a phone which is a phoneme. However, a stimulability assessment show that it is actually a physical articulation disorder. |
| 7. | **Articulation disorder** Child is not stimulable/cannot imitate phones that s/he should be able to at this age | and **Phonological Delay** Phonological simplification processes are observed in the child's speech which are found in younger children's speech |
| 8. | **Articulation disorder** Child is not stimulable/cannot imitate phones that s/he should be able to at this age | and **Consistent Phonological Disorder** Inconsistency of WORD production is <40% Phonological processes observed in the child's speech are NOT found in younger children's speech |
| 9. | **Articulation disorder** Child is not stimulable/cannot imitate phones that s/he should be able to at this age | and **Inconsistent Phonological Disorder** Inconsistency of WORD production is >40% No phonological process may be recognised as words are realised differently on each attempt (no patterns) |

**Table 7.3** Checklist for the assessment of Speech Sound Disorder in bilingual children

| Assessment | Purpose | Level |
|---|---|---|
| Carry out a speech systems examination (an examination of the child's vocal tract) | Rule out *vocal tract abnormality* such as a sub-mucous cleft palate, missing teeth, or unusual bite | Articulation |
| **Home language single-word naming assessment** Name a list of culturally appropriate, high frequency words, balanced for distribution of phones of the home language | Assess the child's ability to use the *range of phonemes* found in the home language *in words* (word initial, word final and within-word syllable initial/final) | Phonological |
| **Repeat a minimum of 10 words from the single-word naming assessment** | Evaluation of the *consistency* of single *word* production | Phonological |
| **Stimulability assessment** Circle any phones produced incorrectly/not on target in words. Ask the child to imitate the sounds as single phones | *Realisation of individual phones* (and/or in CV, VC and CVC structures where these are not real words in any of the child's languages) Differentiates phonological errors (made because the child doesn't yet know where and how to use the phone in words), from phonetic/articulation disorder (where the error is due to the child being unable to physically produce the sound at all, even as a single sound) | Articulation |
| Ask the child to describe a series of culturally appropriate scenes, such as composite pictures. | Evaluation of errors in *connected speech*. | Compare with articulation and phonology errors above AND evaluate suprasegmental aspects of speech including word stress and intonation. |
| Assess for co-morbidity, including: • Listening vocabulary (recognising words) • Naming vocabulary • Language skills • Fluency In both/all languages | Children with Speech Sound Disorder often experience other areas of difficulty. Poor vocabulary will need to be addressed as semantic knowledge triggers selection of phonemes, and children need semantic knowledge to appreciate communication errors when minimal pairs are employed in therapy. | Speech and language systems Interface of vocabulary/ semantics and phonology |
| If the child has sufficient language skills in their additional language: | Carry out the above steps in the additional language in a separate session. | |

## SPEECH SOUND DISORDER: CATEGORISATION

| Physical and Motor:<br>Vocal tract or neurological aetiology | | | PHONOLOGICAL DISORDERS<br>Psycholinguistic: No physical aetiology (idiopathic); hearing impairment such as otitis media with effusion? Genetics? | | |
| --- | --- | --- | --- | --- | --- |
| **Articulation disorder**<br><br>*Cannot imitate sound in isolation*<br><br><br>**12.5% of referred children** | **Dysarthria**<br>*Strength and range of movement, slow or too rapid speech; Intonation disturbed, voice strength affected*<br><br>*Found in clinical sub-groups with a clear medical aetiology, e.g. traumatic brain injury* | **Dyspraxia**<br>*Motor planning errors*<br><br>*Children with motor cortex lesions, like adults, will experience whole body dyspraxia, often affecting speech.*<br>*Developmental verbal dyspraxia (DVD)/ Childhood apraxia of speech (CAS) is extremely rare and controversial. Recommended that inconsistency be ruled out prior to diagnosis* | **Phonological delay**<br><br><br>*Errors found in younger children's speech*<br>**57.5% of referred children** | **Phonological disorder – Consistent**<br><br><br>*Errors NOT found in younger children's speech*<br>**20.6% of referred children** | **Phonological disorder – Inconsistent**<br><br><br>*WORDS produced differently each attempt*<br>**9.4% of referred children** |

**Figure 7.1** Speech Sound Disorder categorisation

*Source*: Adapted from Broomfield and Dodd (2004b)
Note that "Speech Sound Disorder" is an overarching category, not a diagnosis.

## Assessment of Speech Sound Disorder

Most SSDs are idiopathic. That is, there is no known underlying cause. It is important to remember that some children and young people will have SSD associated with an underlying cause such as dysarthria caused by cerebral palsy, or a young person presenting with dyspraxia following a traumatic brain injury. These cases are, however, rare compared with the vast majority of children with SSD.

The main purposes of assessment are:

- To differentiate typical bilingual development from disorder
- To identify the sub-categories of SSD:
  - Articulation disorder, present at sound level and so language is irrelevant; and/or
  - Phonological Delay/Consistent Phonological Disorder/Inconsistent Phonological Disorder
    - Only **one** phonological diagnosis is possible
    - The same *type* of problem will be present (e.g., error patterns not found in younger children's speech for Consistent Phonological Disorder, or inconsistency of word production)
    - Specific error patterns and errors may differ and even contradict across languages, e.g., Stopping in home language but not in English, or fronting in one language but backing in another.
- To identify aims for intervention

Assessment must therefore be carried out in both/all languages, since phonological errors may be different for each language, especially where phones are not shared between the two languages.

## Assessment of hearing

All children with SSD should be referred to Audiology. Not only may hearing impairments be the underlying cause of the child or young person's difficulties, but intermittent or temporary physical disorders such as middle ear infection (otitis media with or without effusion) may be the cause of irritability, lack of attention, loss of balance and other symptoms that affect a child's ability to cooperate with assessment and therapy (NHS 24, 2022).

A child with middle ear infections may also have difficulties hearing and discriminating specific phones due to some frequency bands being attenuated. For this reason, it is help-ful to consider the frequency and loudness of a phone and map this onto the child's audio-gram. The "Speech Banana Chart" is helpful to map the phones of speech onto frequency (Hz) and loudness (dB) (Hill, 2022).

Some children will present with neurological or other permanent hearing impairment. Hearing aids or cochlea implant may be considered. These specialist areas are beyond the remit of this book, but SLTs are usually members of the multi-disciplinary teams assisting families.

## Vocabulary assessment

Since the semantic system interfaces with the phonological system to encode meaning into speech, vocabulary items activate the selection of phoneme. A limited vocabulary may be a significant difficulty for children with SSD. Assessment of word recognition and knowl-edge is therefore helpful when considering the level of breakdown in the speech system.

For young children, adaptations of basic vocabulary lists are available (see *Adaptations in Other Languages* - MacArthur-Bates Communicative Development Inventories) (CDI Advisory Board, 2015).

For all children with SSD, targeting the knowledge of lexical items used in therapy, such as minimal pairs, will ensure that there is strong activation of the semantic system. The use of a word web to visually map semantic and phonological features of an unfamiliar lexical item has long been employed with children (Best et al., 2018).

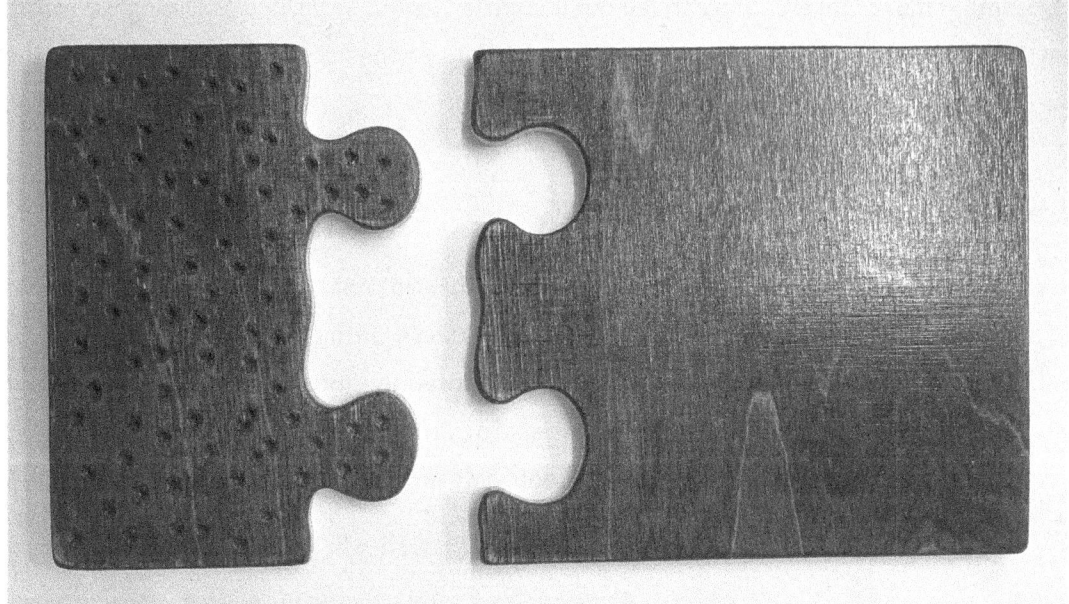

**Figure 7.2** Onset rime wooden jigsaw

*Word web: semantic features*

- **Description**: What does it look like? What parts can you see? How would it feel? What colour(s) can you see? How big is it?
- **Location**: Where would you see this?
- **Function**: What does it do/What sound does it make?

*Word web: phonological features*

- How many syllables (claps/beats) does the word have?
- What is the first sound (onset-rime)?
- How many phones (sounds, *not letters or graphemes*) make up the word?

## Adaptations to word webs for bilingual children

When selecting words for therapy it is important to consider if the child would ever encounter the word in their experience of their community's culture. Examples include cutlery for cultures who eat mainly with their hands and/or flatbreads, and variation in the depiction of foods. It is even worth considering the *brand* and packaging of food and drinks, as young children may only have experience of one particular food brand. When working with Pakistani-heritage children in the north of England, we found that young children recognised the local dairy yoghurt brand and colour of packaging, but not others. This is unsurprising as children as young as three years old have been shown to have high brand awareness (Arnas & Ogul, 2016; Kopelman et al., 2007).

Syllable clapping is important since the largest segmental unit of speech is syllables. However, children from pre-literate cultures may need help to understand this task. We produced a wooden plate with coloured handprints (one hand, two hands and three hands) for children to "clap out" words onto. This tactile approach was highly successful in helping children to understand the concept of syllables and then count the number of hand claps (since clapping hands together leaves no lasting record of how many claps or syllables have been clapped!).

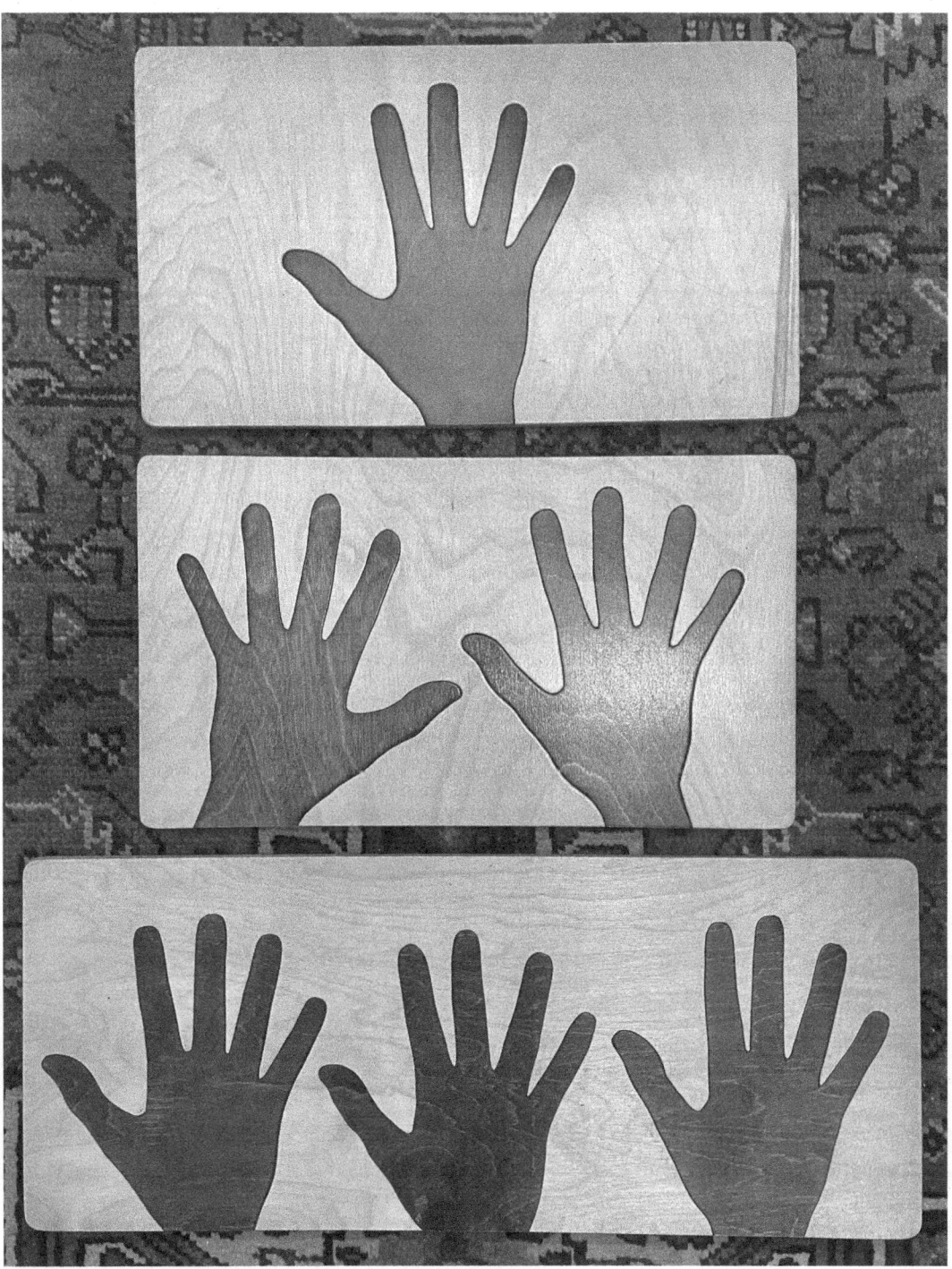

**Figure 7.3** Syllable hand clapping wooden plates

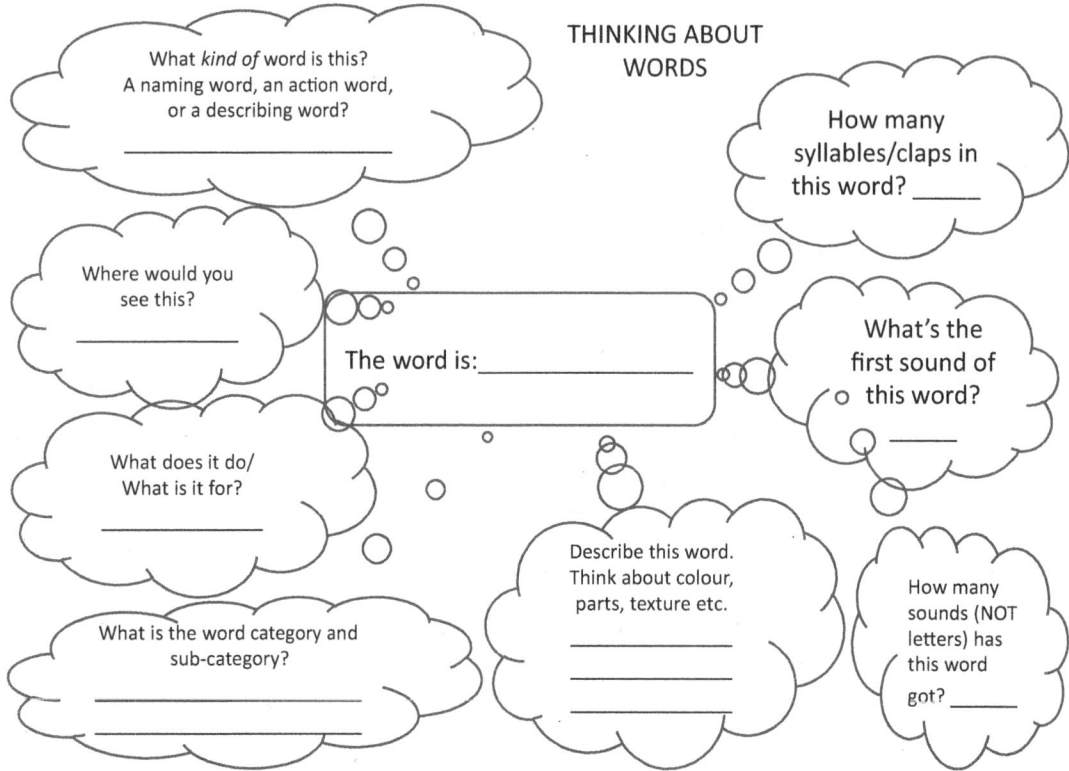

**Figure 7.4** Thinking about words

This may be cheaply reproduced for home practice by getting children to draw around their hands and colour them in, or place their hands in paint and print them onto cards.

Since most young children have not acquired literacy skills, are in the process of doing so, or have no written form for their home language, using articulograms for the first sound (onset) or even sounding out the whole word cannot be usefully completed using printed letters (orthography). Instead, the use of articulograms and/or signs can be helpful. Using resources such as *Bigmouth Sounds* (Hughes & Ramsay, 1994; Ramsay & Hughes, 2012) and *Cued Articulation* (Passy, 2010) are helpful, although for phones not found in English, the clinician will have to adapt these systems and invent their own articulograms and signs (for example, for retroflex sounds in Pakistani-heritage languages). See Figure 7.5.

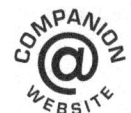

# Checklist for speech assessment of a bilingual child speaking at least one language not shared with the clinician

| 1. | Check the language(s) spoken in the home with the family |
|---|---|
| ❏ | **Look up the languages likely to be spoken by the family** using local statistics, school language surveys and local cultural knowledge. |
| ❏ | **Provide a choice of possible home languages,** such as<br>"Do you speak Mirpuri, Punjabi, Urdu, or another language as well as English?" |
| ❏ | **Check that the language reported matches the language of the professional interpreter** on the pre-session three-way telephone or Telehealth call to the family |
| ❏ | **Research the language(s)**<br>Identify peer-reviewed information on the phonetic and phonological acquisition of the language(s) spoken by the family.<br>Identify any assessments published *where available* |
| ❏ | **Plan the assessment session - 45-60 minutes**<br>Where a published assessment is not available, **identify a set of words likely to be known by young children which can be used as an informal assessment,** including phonemes from normative acquisition data. This should be carried out in collaboration with a professional interpreter with sufficient time to make/adjust resources before the assessment appointment. Take into account any cultural differences. That is, reject words the child may not be familiar with and any words which might be offensive.<br>Discuss technical terms, including "sound" and "word," and how these can be best translated. You should always provide examples to assist with understanding.<br>**Transcribe target words with IPA script.**<br>Plan to assess at least 10 words on two occasions in the assessment session to establish the level of whole word inconsistency production (important for the diagnosis of Inconsistent Phonological Disorder, characterised by high levels of inconsistency of lexical word production)<br>Plan to assess other areas, including language and vocabulary. It is possible that there is co-morbidity, or that the child has other difficulties such as dysfluency that are unrelated to speech sound production.<br>Ask the interpreter to **translate how to greet the family** in home language and transcribe this in IPA script. |
| ❏ | **Greet the family and child in home language**<br>This will welcome the family and signal to the child that home language is acceptable in this setting.<br>Introduce the interpreter, tell the family your name and job title and explain your role. |
| ❏ | **Explain the assessment procedure to the family**<br>**Explain that everything said by anyone in the session will be translated. This includes everything spoken in English into home language, and everything in home language into English. This should include all asides, and comments to the interpreter**<br>Families may be unfamiliar with speech and language therapy and may have very different expectations of assessment.<br>Parent(s)/carers will be able to inform you of any variants in word naming. This may range from codeswitching where words from any of the languages spoken may be employed, through to dialectal variations, and protowords.<br>Explain that the child may need time to name items and that you and the interpreter will help the child and so the family do not have to encourage or name items for the child. |
| ❏ | **Explain what is required to the child/young person**<br>This should be in home language and explain that they can name words any way they wish.<br>Explain that they should say "I don't know" (in home language) if they do not know the name of a picture. |

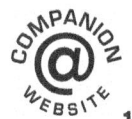
| | |
|---|---|
| ❏ | **Transcribe the child's word naming using IPA script: Include at least 10 words twice**<br><br>An audio or video recording (with appropriate consent) will be helpful for you to check your live transcriptions later and avoid asking the child or young person to repeat the word on multiple occasions. |
| ❏ | **Carry out a stimulability assessment: Imitating single sounds**<br><br>Circle any phones produced incorrectly and ask the child to imitate these.<br><br>It is best to ask the interpreter to model each individual phone.<br><br>If the child cannot imitate phones that they should have acquired by this age then an articulation disorder is present.<br><br>If the child can imitate phones but not use them in words, then a Phonological Delay or disorder is present. |
| ❏ | **Carry out a connected speech assessment**<br><br>Ask the child to describe some culturally appropriate pictures of actions or events.<br><br>Record for later analysis.<br><br>You should observe the same errors as in single-word naming *or more frequent/more severe errors*. |
| ❏ | **Ask parent(s)/carer to rate intelligibility *or carry out other suitable outcome measure***<br><br>Intelligibility ratings are available in many languages.<br><br>See Intelligibility in Context Scale – Multilingual Children's Speech (McLeod et al., 2012):<br><br>www.csu.edu.au/research/multilingual-speech/ics |
| ❏ | **Carry out a speech systems examination**<br><br>Examination of the vocal tract, bite, elevation of the velum and ruling out physical causes of speech disorder should be carried out.<br><br>See the **Speech Systems Examination Form.**<br><br>**NB.** Carefully observe infection control measures and only complete where safe to do so. |
| ❏ | **Debriefing session**<br><br>Discussion of the child's speech should be undertaken with the interpreter.<br><br>Consider that the child may have used an alternative but appropriate word to name items.<br><br>The interpreter will be able to comment on the child or young person's intelligibility in home language. |
| ❏ | **Analyse the data**<br><br>If inconsistency of word production is >50%, plan an inconsistency assessment<br><br>If inconsistency of word production is <40%:<br><br>• Circle any errors/differences<br>• Describe any systematic errors<br>• Compare to normative data on simplification patterns<br>• Only apply normative data where the child is comparable (see notes)<br>• Reach a provisional diagnosis<br><br>Scores of 40–50% are borderline and it is recommended that an inconsistency assessment is completed. |
| ❏ | **In a separate session** assess the child's additional/other language(s) in the same way.<br><br>Remember to use any normative data (such as phonological process age norms) as a guide but recall that bilingual children will take longer to acquire two or more languages compared to the monolingual's single language – the bilingual is not two monolinguals in one! |

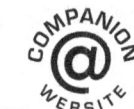

| | |
|---|---|
| ❏ | **Consider a diagnosis**<br><br>Articulation disorder will be the same across both/all languages, since this relates to the physical production of phones.<br><br>A Speech Sound Disorder will **not** be present in only one language.<br><br>Phonological Delay, Consistent Phonological Disorder and Inconsistent Phonological Disorder will be present in both/all languages. However, the surface patterns may differ in each language. |
| ❏ | **Onward referral(s)**<br><br>If a child or young person does present with any type of Speech Sound Disorder, then a referral to Audiology should be made. If a hearing impairment is present, the SLT should liaise with the Audiologist to better understand the implications for therapy, for example high frequency loss affecting fricative development.<br><br>Any physical abnormalities discovered in the speech systems examination should be referred to the appropriate multidisciplinary team, such as Ear, Nose and Throat and/or the Regional Cleft Lip and Palate Team. |
| ❏ | **Assessment report and recommendations for intervention**<br><br>A full written report of the assessment findings should be written. All recommendations should be based on the evidence-base and not be limited by rationing or availability of care, even if you are aware of these limiting factors.<br><br>For bilingual children with confirmed Speech Sound Disorder, recommendations must include:<br><br>**"Intervention should be carried out with the assistance of an interpreter or classroom assistant who speaks [language(s)]"**<br><br>**"Therapy aims should be completed in the home language prior to English"**<br><br>and, depending on the parent(s)'/carers' language abilities:<br><br>**"An interpreter should be present in order to ensure that the child/young person's parent(s)/carer is able to engage in the therapy process and so that they can be fully involved in any decision making by providing informed parental consent"** |
| ❏ | **Provide the parent(s)/carer with translation of the assessment report**<br><br>For parent(s)/carers who are highly literate, a written translation may be helpful. This should be carried out by a translator, since electronic translation apps and website may transmit confidential patient data outside the country and breach Data Protection legislation.<br><br>For most parents, an audio version in home language may be much more useful. In this case, invite the parent(s)/carer to a meeting and ask the interpreter to translate the report and ask parent(s)/carer to record this on their mobile phone for later reference and to share with the extended family if they so wish.<br><br>Also provide a written English language report so that parent(s)/carer can share the report with other professionals.<br><br>Discuss any questions the parent(s)/carer may have and request consent to share the report with the wider multidisciplinary team, such as the GP, Special Educational Needs and Disability Coordinator, teacher, and bilingual classroom assistant. |

## Notes on the checklist

Language(s) spoken are often misreported by referring agents, and many parent(s)/carers may state a language that they think you may be familiar with, rather than providing a more accurate answer. Others report the high-status variety of the language family, while actually speaking a related, lower status language. Some families may even deny using a home language, as they have absorbed the myth that home language use will slow down the acquisition of the language of learning (such as English, Welsh or Gaelic in the UK).

## Offer a choice of languages

Ensure that you offer a choice of languages, including all the languages within a particular community. For example, ask Pakistani-heritage families, "Do you speak Mirpuri, Punjabi, Urdu, or another language?"

## Identify the inventory and any developmental data for the language(s)

It is important to know which phonemes make up the contrastive system. These data are usually found in research papers. However, if there is no reliable data from a peer-reviewed journal or book chapter, the therapist may have to use more informal sources of information. Other sources of information are experts in language. Consider contacting:

- Academics working in linguistics at a local university
- Therapists who speak the language
- Therapists, professionals, or researchers in the home/heritage country

Recall that many referrals list the wrong language, parent(s)/carers may report a high-status language rather than the actual language used in the home, and you may need to identify the correct "dialect" (or more likely separate, but related language).

There are increasingly books and research papers available which describe the phonology, phonetic inventory, use of tones, and other suprasegmental phonological features (where present). These may be available through your employer, a professional organisation, or a university library.

There are also some examples of speech sound screen and assessments in languages other than English.

## Monolingual acquisition data is likely to differ from bilingual acquisition data and should not be applied to bilingual children unmodified

Where bilingual acquisition data is unavailable, use monolingual acquisition data/phonological processes **descriptively**. Normative data on the age of acquisition of phones and phonemes, and the suppression/elimination of phonological processes will typically be later for bilingual children and may occur in a different order.

## Information on the phonology of languages other than English (LOTE)

Professional bodies have lists and/or links to data on the speech sound acquisition and phonological processes for many LOTE.

- RCSLT, UK: www.rcslt.org/members/clinical-guidance/bilingualism/bilingualism-learning#section-11
- ASHA, US: www.asha.org/practice/multicultural/Phono/

## Features which may be unfamiliar to English monolingual therapists

Most SLTs are English speakers in the UK and US. This cultural bias means that features of languages other than English may be surprising, especially if the therapist has not encountered a particular language previously.

*Contrast*

The role of the phonological system is to provide a system of contrasts so that different word meanings may be encoded efficiently and transmitted to the listener. In English phonology, the main contrasts in consonants are signalled by three features:

- Voice (voiceless or voiced)
- Place: the position of the constriction, occlusion, or approximation within the vocal tract
- Manner (nasal, plosive, fricative, approximant, affricate, etc.)

In Mirpuri, a Pakistani-heritage language, there is a three-way contrast for the first contrast, voicing:

- Voiceless and Aspirated, e.g., "flower" /pʰʊl /
- Voiceless unaspirated, e.g., bridge /pʊl /
- Fully voiced, e.g., "lips"/"mouth" /bʊl /

English also adds aspiration to word initial plosives, but the aspirated and unaspirated allophones are considered to be variants of the same phoneme, as in "paper"/ˈpʰeɪ.pə /.

In contrast, Spanish employs only voiced and voiceless plosives. None of them are aspirated (Wayland, 2019).

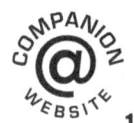

Place may also be important in ways not employed by the English phonological system of contrast. For example, English has no dental consonants, and to produce an alveolar plosive with dentalisation would be perceived as a distortion (a "lisp"). Mirpuri speakers would perceive the *lack* of dentalisation as an error for words such as "milk" / d̪ud̪ / (Stow & Pert, 2020).

## Speech Systems Examination

## Purpose

This is a brief, routine, screening assessment of articulators to identify areas for further investigation. More detailed investigations are available (see for example Sell et al., 1999) This speech systems examination is for use as a first screening tool and is appropriate to use with all children identified as needing speech and language therapy input for Speech Sound Disorder.

## Equipment

**NB.** Infection control equipment should be used (Consider cytomegalovirus) (Zuhair et al., 2019): Gloves, tissues, spatula, pocket torch, small mirror.

**NB.** Potential aerosol generating procedure - Take appropriate precautions! (See Chacon et al., 2021). Medical mask, gloves, ventilation, hand washing, and testing.

| First name(s): | | Last name: | |
|---|---|---|---|
| Date of birth: | / / | Age: YY;MM | ; |
| NHS / ID number: | | | |
| Date of assessment: | / /20 | Assessed by: | |
| Clinic/Site: | | | |

| | Structure | Description | Tick | Comments |
|---|---|---|---|---|
| 1. | **Lips** | Normal | | Within normal limits |
| | | Cleft lip | | |
| 2. | **Teeth** | Normal | | Within normal limits |
| | | Class I Malocclusion | | Bite appropriate but teeth rotated or crooked |
| | | Class II Malocclusion | | Upper teeth stick out past lower teeth ("overbite") |
| | | Class III Malocclusion | | Lower teeth stick out past upper teeth ("underbite") |
| | | Open Bite | | Central gap when teeth are together often caused by prolonged dummy /bottle/ feeder cup use |
| | | Missing or decayed dentition | | |

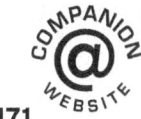

|  | Structure | Description | Tick | Comments |
|---|---|---|---|---|
| 3. | **Tongue** Size in relation to dental arches | Appropriate | | |
| | | Too large | | |
| | | Too small | | |
| | | Tight lingual frenulum | | Can touch alveolar ridge Cannot touch alveolar ridge |
| 4. | **Hard Palate** | Normal | | |
| | | Palatal contour – High arch | | |
| | | Palatal contour – Flat arch | | |
| | | Cleft/fistula | | |
| | | Notch present | | |
| 5. | **Palatopharyngeal mechanism** | Normal soft palate/velum | | |
| | | Cleft soft palate | | |
| | | Normal uvular | | |
| | | Cleft or bifid uvular | | Indicative of submucous cleft |
| | | Bluish or white line/patches | | Indicative of submucous cleft |

|  | Observation | Tick if observed | |
|---|---|---|---|
| 1. | Mouth breathing | | Habitual even without a cold? |
| 2. | Drooling | | |
| 3. | Hyponasal speech | | No air released from nose (sounds like a blocked nose due to a cold) |
| 4. | Hypernasal speech | | Air escapes from nose even on oral sounds such as vowels. Check with a small mirror under the nose when saying vowels (misting indicates air released) |
| 5. | Mixed resonance | | Evidence of both hypo- and hypernasal speech |

| Tick | Outcome and action |
|---|---|
| | 1. No action. Discharge or standard speech sound treatment is appropriate. |
| | 2. Refer to the local specialist speech and language therapist for further investigation. Please complete a *full* DEAP assessment (Dodd et al., 2002) or equivalent. |
| | 3. Refer to the Regional Cleft Lip and Palate Network |

**File in *Assessments* section of speech and language therapy case notes.**

## Why the application of monolingual normative data, including phonological process age of elimination is misleading

Grech and Dodd (2008, p. 169) state that "Comparison of a bilingual child's developmental profile with that of monolingual children could lead to misdiagnosis." This is because a bilingual child cannot be compared to the monolingual acquisition data for *either of their two languages*. The child is not two monolingual speakers rolled into one.

## Applying phonological process age norms across languages

SLTs may be tempted to apply normative data from one language to another, especially when the phonological processes are the same. This would be an error, as different phonological systems have different acquisition rates. This is demonstrated when comparing normative data across languages.

## Phonological processes are eliminated at different ages across languages

Consider the following phonological processes. The first column of age norms shows the age at which 90% of children eliminate the simplification pattern in English, whilst the

**Table 7.4** A comparison of the age when phonological processes are suppressed for English versus Mirpuri-speaking children

| Phonological process | Age at which 90% of children eliminate the phonological process/simplification pattern in English (UK) | Age at which children eliminate the phonological process/simplification pattern in Mirpuri |
| --- | --- | --- |
| Stopping<br>*fricative replaced by a plosive* | 3;5<br>e.g., "van"/**væn**/➜[bæn] | 5;5<br>e.g., "clean"/sɑːf/➜[tɑː] |
| Fronting<br>*Produced more anterior in the vocal tract* | 3;11<br>e.g., "egg"/eɡ/➜[ed] | 4;11<br>e.g., "clothes"/kʊkəɽi/➜[tʊtəli] |
| Context Sensitive Voicing<br>*Pre-vocalic addition of voicing or post-vocalic devoicing* | <3;0<br>e.g., "pram"/pɹæm/➜[bæm] | 4;11<br>e.g., "banana"/kela/➜[gela] |
| Weak syllable deletion | 3;11<br>e.g., "tomato"/təˈmɑ.təʊ/➜[mɑ.təʊ] | 5;5<br>e.g., "chicken"/kʊkəɽi/➜[ɽi] |
| Reduplication | 2-year-old sample<br>e.g., "tiger"/ˈtaɪ.ɡə/➜[taɪtaɪ] | 4;11<br>e.g., "milk" / ɖ ʊɖ /➜[ɖ ʊɖ u] |
| Assimilation<br>*Influence of another phoneme in the target word* | 2-year-old sample<br>e.g., "yellow"/ˈje.ləʊ/➜[leləʊ] | 3;5<br>e.g., "key" / d͡ʒabi/➜[babi] |
| *Intrusive consonant* | Unusual/disordered process | 6;11<br>e.g., "clean"/sɑːf/ ➜ [stɑːf] |
| *De-retroflex* | No retroflex phonemes in English phonology | 5;5<br>e.g., "flour"/aʈa/ ➜ [ata] |
| *De-dentalisation* | No dental plosives in English phonology | 5;5<br>e.g., "milk" / ɖ uɖ / ➜ [dud] |

(Adapted from Dodd et al., 2003; Stow & Pert, 2020)

second column of age norms show the age at which Pakistani-heritage children growing up in England eliminated the pattern in their home language, Mirpuri. As you can see, there are differences across the two languages.

This illustrates that the same phonological processes are eliminated at different ages across languages.

The bottom three rows illustrate that some phonological processes are unique to that language's phonology and may be an age-appropriate or delayed phonological process for one language (for example, intrusive consonant in Mirpuri), whereas in another language this would be considered a disordered phonological process (English).

## Interaction of two languages and the impact on phonology

Typically developing bilingual children may have patterns in one or both of their languages not seen in the speech of monolingual speakers. For example, a Mirpuri-English-speaking child was observed to have word final nasal stopping in her English:

e.g., "crown"/kɹaʊn/➜ [kɹaʊn**d**] (Holm et al., 1999, p. 283)

This process was observed in the speech of over half (18/35) of the bilingual children assessed. This delayed process, observed in younger children from the same community, would be regarded as a disordered process if observed in the speech of a monolingual English-speaking child. However, for this child, her stopping in Urdu was of fricative and (deaffrication) of affricates.

Similarly, the bilingual children in this study simplified clusters using a schwa rather than omitting a segment. For example, "flower"/ˈflaʊ.wə/➜ [fəlaʊwə]. Although occasionally observed in the speech of English monolingual children, it was observed in all 35 bilingual children.

## Same phonological diagnosis, different surface patterns in each language

*Articulation disorder*

Since we have only one vocal tract, articulation disorder (assessed by stimulability of single phones) is evident across both/all languages. Producing a single phone has no meaning and is not subject to phonological processes at sound level (or in consonant + vowel (CV), vowel + consonant (VC) or consonant + vowel + consonant (CVC) combinations) **provided** these have no lexical meaning in either language.

**Table 7.5** Speech Sound Disorder diagnoses and features

| | |
|---|---|
| SPEECH SOUND DISORDERS | Category level label used to discuss ALL speech sound pathology |
| Articulation disorder | Error(s) on the production of single **phones** (sounds in isolation), with the resulting phone described as a *distortion* (as it is not a phoneme of that language), and/or errors at CV, VC or CVC combinations **provided** such combinations are *not words in any of the languages the child speaks*. |
| Articulation disorder with phonological implications | This is the same as Articulation Disorder. However, the error **results in another phoneme in that language**, rather than a distortion (a phone that is not in that language is produced as the error).<br><br>Such errors are often mistaken for phonological processes if a stimulability assessment is not undertaken. |
| PHONOLOGICAL DISORDERS | Category label for all phonological pathology<br>Errors, omissions and/or substitutions caused by a lack of contrast, or faulty mapping of meaning onto the contrastive system (phonological system)<br>Occurs at **word level** (and phrase and utterance level)<br>The child is stimulable for phones at sound level but fails to use them at word level.<br>Assessment is essential in both/all languages as surface patterns may differ across languages.<br>The underlying phonological subgroup, listed below, will be evident in both/all languages, although different phonemes may be affected. |
| Phonological Delay | Simplification/phonological processes are observed in younger children's speech.<br>Note that:<br>1. For bilingual/multilingual children the therapist would need to know the normative developmental data for:<br>  a. Monolingual acquisition of the home language<br>  b. Monolingual acquisition of the mainstream language<br>  c. Bilingual acquisition context<br>The normative data for the order of acquisition is likely to be similar in all contexts, but the age of acquisition may differ.<br>These data may not exist if the language(s) have not been researched from a speech sound acquisition perspective.<br>2. "Delay" does **not** imply that the child will resolve these difficulties without speech and language therapy input. Problems are likely to persist if left untreated.<br>3. "Phonological delay" refers to the speech **patterns**; it *never* becomes phonological disorder, despite the age of the child or young person. |
| Consistent Phonological Disorder | Simplification/phonological processes are unusual and **not observed** in younger children's speech. They are atypical at any age.<br>Note that for bilingual children:<br>1. Disordered processes may only be defined in relation to delayed processes. Therefore, normative data is required on typical versus atypical speech sound development in the language(s) the child speaks.<br>2. Bilingual children may have features in one or both languages which would be considered unusual in a monolingual speaker (Hua & Dodd, 2006). |
| Inconsistent Phonological Disorder | The child produces **words** differently on each occasion and cannot reliably map meaning onto word templates.<br>There is in effect, no phonological system and so any apparent phonological processes are an illusion (they would change if you asked the child to name the word list again).<br>Note that for bilingual children:<br>The Core Vocabulary Approach (McIntosh & Dodd, 2009) utilises words that the child is likely to say in their everyday lives. For most children, these items are likely to be in their home language, as children spend longer at home than in school at any age. |

*Phonological disorders*

"Phonological disorders" is a category of Speech Sound Disorders referring to word-level errors, omissions, and substitutions. This confusion includes "Phonological Delay."

## Planning intervention for a bilingual child with Speech Sound Disorder

## Treatment intensity (Dose)

As with all care pathways for bilingual children, treatment is likely to take at least double the time compared to that for a monolingual child who shares a (mainstream) language (such as English) with the therapist in order to achieve the same outcomes.

If the same amount of time is allocated, the bilingual child is highly likely to have poorer outcomes since actual input will be significantly less than for a monolingual child, considering the need to work alongside an interpreter, identify normative data in languages other than English, and assess, diagnose, and treat a Speech Sound Disorder in a language the therapist is unfamiliar with. Failure to allocate double the time for an episode of care is a clear example of institutional racism.

## Articulation disorder

Therapy focusing on the placement of articulators (Secord et al., 2007), visual feedback using a therapy mirror, articulograms (diagrams of how to place articulators, such as the "Bigmouth Sounds" (Ramsay & Hughes, 2012), and signing, such as "Cued Articulation" (Passy, 2010), is implemented. Drill work, that is, many tens or even hundreds of repetitions per therapy session, may be required before a child or young person can consistently produce a phone on demand.

Articulation therapy may be required prior to working at word level. This is particularly true for children who have articulation disorder with phonological implications. To work on an apparent phonological process which is actually caused by an articulation error would likely result in a poor outcome.

Most intervention resources target the phones of English. Many languages contain other phones and different important contrasts. These should be noted and assessed in the stimulability assessment. The SLT should also consider adapting therapy resources to include these phones. An example shown in Figure 7.5 is a Bigmouth Sound articulogram for a voiced retroflex tap (adapted by Hammad, 2022 from Ramsay & Hughes, 2012).

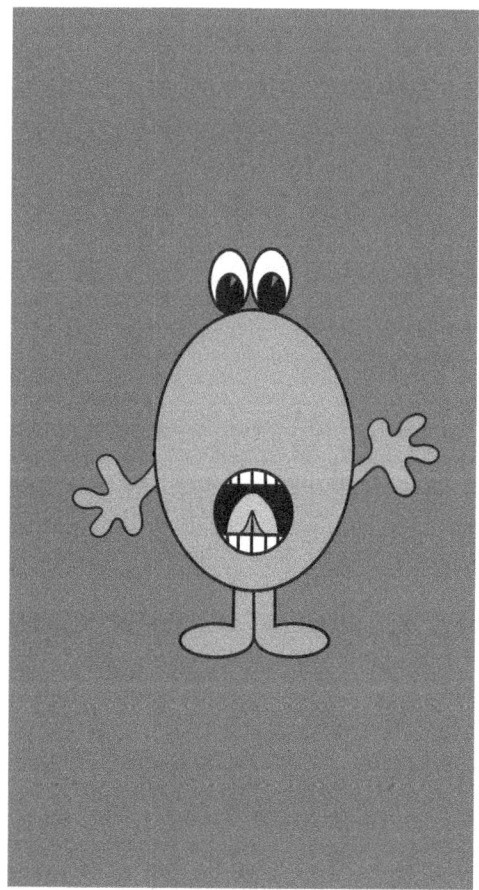

**Figure 7.5** Bigmouth Sound Picture (Articulogram) adapted for a voiced retroflex tap (Hammad, 2022 adapted from Hughes & Ramsay, 1994; Ramsay & Hughes, 2012)

Resources which include video animations of all the phones on the International Phonetic Alphabet chart based on ultrasound and MRI may be found on the Internet. "Seeing Speech" (Lawson et al., 2018) allows the therapist to ear-train for phones that may not be in your own language and assist in the development of appropriate placement cues for the child.

## Phonological Delay and Consistent Phonological Disorder

Unlike articulatory approaches, phonological therapy should help the child to real-ise that the selection of the incorrect phoneme leads to a change in meaning for the listener. Common approaches cited by 366 speech-language pathologists in the US (Brumbaugh & Smit, 2013) included Phonological awareness, Minimal pairs, and Cycles (Hodson, 1983).

For bilingual children, adapting these approaches to a language other than English will involve knowledge of both the *meaning* of lexical items and the *phonological form* of lexical items.

It is taken for granted by people who speak a literate language that "dictionary access" to lexical items is natural and universal. It is thought that exposure to written language (orthography) changes the cognitive processes of the brain (Kerckhove, 1986). For speakers of languages with no written form, this access cannot be taken for granted. Clinically, this may mean that an interpreter who is able to, say, provide a word list of words starting with /s/ in English (a language they are literate in), may find the same task much more challenging in their non-literate home language (or language which has a radically different script from the Roman script of most European languages).

This was the case when constructing a speech sound screen in Mirpuri, a pre-literate Pakistani-heritage language (Stow & Pert, 1998). In order to get around this, it is helpful for the therapist to identify phonemes in the language and ask if any words contain these sounds. This phonemic cueing can be helpful when identifying words for therapy targets. Minimal pairs, or near minimal pairs can then be identified by changing one phoneme. The therapist will need to decide if the words identified are concrete (able to be drawn, or a photograph taken of the object or activity) and suitable for young children.

In common with all children with Consistent Phonological Disorder, the error patterns are by definition, unusual. Bespoke minimal pairs or lexical items containing the target phoneme, contrasting with the phoneme produced by the child in the error pattern would need to be identified.

## Inconsistent Phonological Disorder (IPD)

Since the intervention for IPD is not based on phonological processes or specific phonemes, but rather the consistent production of words (even if they are not on target), it is relatively simple to adapt the Core Vocabulary Therapy approach (Dodd et al., 2004). Target words simply need to be those the child is likely to use in the course of their everyday life in the home language.

## Summary

The assessment, diagnosis and treatment of Speech Sound Disorders is a central role of the SLT. For bilingual children, or those speaking languages other than English, the challenge is to differentiate diversity from disorder. There are a far greater number of languages where the phonetic inventory and phonological contrastive system have been described in the literature in the last few decades than were previously available. Innovations such as online

IPA charts with sound and animation make it possible for therapists to become familiar with phonemes that may not feature in their own language. Other features of contrast, including lexical tone, and, to monolingual English speakers, unfamiliar ways of signalling meaning contrast, such as three way aspirated/voiceless/voiced contrasts need to be noted and explored.

Intervention for phonological disorders (including Phonological Delay) *must* involve assessment and treatment in the home language(s). Intervention does not generalise from say English to the home language (except for non-phonological errors, that is Articulation Disorder). This is because phonology is the mapping of a particular language lexicon onto a language-specific encoding system, the phonology of that language.

# References

American Speech-Hearing Association (ASHA). (2020). *Speech disorders- articulation and phonology. incidence and prevalence*. Retrieved September 6, 2020, from www.asha.org/PRPSpecificTopic.asp x?folderid=8589935321&section=Incidence_and_Prevalence

Arnas, Y. A., Tas, I., & Ogul, I. G. (2016). The development of brand awareness in young children: How do young children recognize brands? *International Journal of Consumer Studies, 40*, 536–542. https://doi.org/10.1111/ijcs.12298

Best, W., Hughes, L. M., Masterson, J., Thomas, M., Fedor, A., Roncoli, S., . . . Kapikian, A. (2018). Intervention for children with word-finding difficulties: A parallel group randomised control trial. *International Journal of Speech Language Pathology, 20*, 708–719. https://doi.org/10.1080/17549507.2017.1348541

Broomfield, J., & Dodd, B. (2004a). The nature of referred subtypes of primary speech disability. *Child Language Teaching and Therapy, 20*, 135–151. https://doi.org/10.1191%2F0265659004ct267oa

Broomfield, J., & Dodd, B. (2004b). Children with speech and language disability: Caseload characteristics. *International Journal of Language & Communication Disorders, 39*(3), 303–324. https://doi.org/10.1080/13682820310001625589

Brosseau-Lapré, F., & Roepke, E. (2019). Speech errors and phonological awareness in children ages four and five years with and without speech sound disorder. *Journal of Speech, Language, and Hearing Research, 62*(9), 3276–3289. https://doi.org/10.1044/2019_JSLHR-S-17-0461

Brumbaugh, K., & Smit, A. (2013). Treating children ages three to six who have speech sound disorder: A survey. *Language, Speech & Hearing Services in Schools (Online), 44*, 306–319. https://doi.org/10.1044/0161-1461(2013/12-0029)

Carr, P. (2013). English intonation. In P. Carr (Ed.), *English phonetics and phonology: An introduction* (2nd ed., pp. 107–125). Blackwell. ISBN: 978-1-4051-3454-5

CDI Advisory Board. (2015). *MacArthur-Bates CDI: Adaptations in other languages. Adaptations, not translations!* Stanford University. Retrieved March 30, 2022, from http://www.mb-cdi.stanford.edu/adaptations.html

Chacon, A. M., Nguyen, D. D., McCabe, P., & Madill, C. (2021). Aerosol-generating behaviours in speech pathology clinical practice: A systematic literature review. *PLoS One, 16*, e0250308. https://doi.org/10.1371/journal.pone.0250308.

Dodd, B., Crosbie, S., & Holm, A. (2004). *Core vocabulary: Intervention for children with inconsistent speech disorder, CD-ROM*. Perinatal Research Centre, The University of Queensland, Australia.

Dodd, B., Holm, A., Crosbie, S., & McCormack, P. (2005). Differential diagnosis of phonological disorders. In B. Dodd (Ed.), *Differential diagnosis and treatment of children with speech disorder* (2nd ed., pp. 44–70). Whurr.

Dodd, B., Holm, A., Hua, Z., & Crosbie, S. (2003). Phonological development: A normative study of British English-speaking children. *Clinical Linguistics and Phonology, 17*(8), 617–643. https://doi.org/https://doi.org/10.1080/0269920031000111348

Dodd, B., Holm, A., Hua, Z., Crosbie, S., & Broomfield, J. (2006). English phonology: Acquisition and disorder. In Z. Hua, & B. Dodd (Eds.), *Phonological development and disorders in children: A multilingual perspective*. Multilingual Matters.

Dodd, B., Hua, Z., Crosbie, S., Holm, A., & Ozanne, A. (2002). *Diagnostic evaluation of articulation and phonology*. Psychological Corporation.

Eadie, P., Morgan, A., Ukoumunne, O. C., Ttofari Eecen, K., Wake, M., & Reilly, S. (2015). Speech sound disorder at 4 years: Prevalence, comorbidities, and predictors in a community cohort of children. *Developmental Medicine & Child Neurology*, 57(6), 578-584. https://doi.org/10.1111/dmcn.12635

Fernald, A., Marchman, V. A., & Weisleder, A. (2013). SES differences in language processing skill and vocabulary are evident at 18 months. *Developmental Science*, 16(2), 234-248. https://doi.org/10.1111/desc.12019

Grech, H., & Dodd, B. (2008). Phonological acquisition in Malta: A bilingual language learning context. *International Journal of Bilingualism*, 12(3), 155-171. https://doi.org/10.1177/1367006908098564

Hammad, R. (2022). *Bigmouth: Voiced retroflex tap articulogram illustration*. Adapted from Hughes, S., & Ramsay, N. (1994). *Bigmouth sound pack*. STASS Publications.

Hesketh, A., Adams, C., Nightingale, C., & Hall, R. (2000). Phonological awareness therapy and articulatory training approaches for children with phonological disorders: A comparative outcome study. *International Journal of Language & Communication Disorders*, 35(3), 337-354. https://doi.org/10.1080/136828200410618

Hill, V. (2022). *Patient information: Speech banana chart*. Centre for Hearing and Balance, University Hospitals Coventry and Warwickshire NHS Trust. www.uhcw.nhs.uk/download/clientfiles/files/Patient%20Information%20Leaflets/Clinical%20Diagnostic%20Services/Audiology/117639_Speech_Banana_Chart_(2025)_May_2018.pdf

Hodson, B. (1983). A facilitative approach for remediation of a child's profoundly unintelligible phonological system. *Topics in Language Disorders*, 3, 24-34. https://psycnet.apa.org/doi/10.1097/00011363-198303000-00006

Holm, A., Dodd, B., Stow, C., & Pert, S. (1999). Identification and differential diagnosis of phonological disorder in bilingual children. *Language Testing*, 16, 271-292. https://doi.org/10.1177%2F026553229901600303

Hua, Z., & Dodd, B. (Eds.). (2006). *Phonological development and disorders in children*. Multilingual Matters.

Hughes, S., & Ramsay, N. (1994). *Bigmouth sound pack*. STASS Publications.

Hussain, Q., Proctor, M., Harvey, M., & Demuth, K. (2020). Punjabi (Lyallpuri variety). *Journal of the International Phonetic Association*, 50, 282-297. https://doi.org/10.1017/S0025100319000021

Kerckhove, D. D. (1986). Alphabetic literacy and brain processes. *Visible Language*, 20, 274-293. https://doi.org/10.1007/978-94-009-2778-0_6

Kopelman, C. A., Roberts, L. M., & Adab, P. (2007). Advertising of food to children: Is brand logo recognition related to their food knowledge, eating behaviours and food preferences? *Journal of Public Health (Oxford, England)*, 29, 358-367. https://doi.org/10.1093/pubmed/fdm067

Lawson, E., Stuart-Smith, J., Scobbie, J. M., & Nakai, S. (2018). *Seeing speech: An articulatory web resource for the study of Phonetics*. University of Glasgow. Retrieved March 30, 2022 www.seeingspeech.ac.uk.

Li, C. N., & Thompson, S. A. (1977). The acquisition of tone in Mandarin-speaking children. *Journal of Child Language*, 4, 185-199. https://doi.org/10.1017/S0305000900001598

Marshall, J., Harding, S., & Roulstone, S. (2017). Language development, delay and intervention-the views of parents from communities that speech and language therapy managers in England consider to be under-served. *International Journal of Language & Communication Disorders*, 52(4), 489-500. https://doi.org/10.1111/1460-6984.12288

McIntosh, B., & Dodd, B. (2009). Evaluation of core vocabulary intervention for treatment of inconsistent phonological disorder: Three treatment case studies. *Child Language Teaching and Therapy*, 25, 9-29. https://doi.org/10.1177/0265659008100811

McLeod, S., Harrison, L. J., & McCormack, J. (2012). The intelligibility in context scale: Validity and reliability of a subjective rating measure. *Journal of Speech, Language, and Hearing Research*, 55(2), 648-656. https://doi.org/10.1044/1092-4388(2011/10-0130)

Morgan, P. L., Hammer, C. S., Farkas, G., Hillemeier, M. M., Maczuga, S., Cook, M., & Morano, S. (2016). Who receives speech/language services by five years of age in the United States? *American Journal of Speech-Language Pathology*, 25(2), 183-199. https://doi.org/10.1044/2015_ajslp-14-0201

Naeem, K., Filippi, R., Periche-Tomas, E., Papageorgiou, A., & Bright, P. (2018). The importance of socioeconomic status as a modulator of the bilingual advantage in cognitive ability. *Frontiers in Psychology*, 9, 1818. https://doi.org/10.3389/fpsyg.2018.01818

Nancollis, A., Lawrie, B.-A., & Dodd, B. (2005). Phonological awareness intervention and the acquisition of literacy skills in children from deprived social backgrounds. *Language, Speech, and Hearing Services in Schools*, 36(4), 325-335. https://doi.org/10.1044/0161-1461(2005/032)

NHS 24. (2022). *Middle ear infection (otitis media)*. NHS Inform. www.nhsinform.scot/illnesses-and-conditions/ears-nose-and-throat/middle-ear-infection-otitis-media

Passy, J. (2010). *Cued articulation: Consonants and vowels* (Rev. ed.). ACER Press.

Ramsay, N., & Hughes, S. (2012). *Bigmouth sounds: App for iPhone/iPad/iTouch*. Vox Aux. www.voxaux.com/bigmouth

Secord, W. A., Boyce, S. E., Fox, R. A., Donohue, J. S., & Shine, R. E. (2007). *Eliciting sounds: techniques and strategies for clinicians* (2nd ed.). Delmar Cengage Learning.

Sell, D., Harding, A., & Grunwell, P. (1999). GOS.SP.ASS.'98: An assessment for speech disorders associated with cleft palate and/or velopharyngeal dysfunction (revised). *International Journal of Language & Communication Disorders, 34*(1), 17–33. https://doi.org/10.1080/136828299247595

So, L. K. H. (2006). Cantonese phonological development: Normal and disordered. In Z. Hua & B. Dodd (Eds.), *Phonological development and disorders in children: A multilingual perspective* (pp. 109–134). Multilingual Matters. ISBN 1-85359-889-5.

Stow, C. & Dodd, B. (2005). A survey of bilingual children referred for investigation of communication disorders: A comparison with monolingual children referred in one area in England. *Journal of Multilingual Communication Disorders, 3*(1), 1–23. https://doi.org/10.1080/14769670400009959.

Stow, C., & Pert, S. (1998). The development of a bilingual phonology assessment. *International Journal of Language & Communication Disorders, 33*, 338–342. https://doi.org/10.3109/13682829809179447.

Stow, C., & Pert, S. (2020). *Bilingual Speech Sound Screen (BiSSS) for children with a Pakistani heritage background speaking Mirpuri, Punjabi or Urdu as a mother tongue in the UK*. The University of Manchester. https://www.estore.manchester.ac.uk/product-catalogue/faculty-of-biology-medicine-and-health/school-of-health-sciences/bilingual-speech-sound-screen-bisss/bilingual-speech-sound-screen-bisss

Waring, R., & Knight, R. (2013). How should children with speech sound disorders be classified? A review and critical evaluation of current classification systems. *International Journal of Language & Communication Disorders, 48*(1), 25–40. https://doi.org/10.1111/j.1460-6984.2012.00195.x

Wayland, R. (2019). *Phonetics: A practical introduction*. Cambridge University Press.

Webb, A. N., Hao, W., & Hong, P. (2013). The effect of tongue-tie division on breastfeeding and speech articulation: A systematic review. *International Journal of Pediatric Otorhinolaryngology, 77*(5), 635–646. https://doi.org/10.1016/j.ijporl.2013.03.008.

Wren, Y. (2019, August 8–9). How do we identify children whose speech problems are unlikely to resolve? In *Ask the experts: Child speech sound disorder: Special edition of Bulletin*. Royal College of Speech and Language Therapists.

Zuhair, M., Smit, G. S. A., Wallis, G., Jabbar, F., Smith, C., Devleesschauwer, B., & Griffiths, P. (2019). Estimation of the worldwide seroprevalence of cytomegalovirus: A systematic review and meta-analysis. *Reviews in Medical Virology, 29*, e2034. https://doi.org/10.1002/rmv.2034

# AUGMENTATIVE AND ALTERNATIVE COMMUNICATION

## LIZZIE SADIKU, KATHERINE SMALL AND SUZANNE MARTIN

DOI: 10.4324/9781003125563-8

# Augmentative and Alternative Communication (AAC) in a bilingual context

Katherine Small, Lizzie Sadiku and Suzanne Martin are AAC Consultants at Ace Centre, a national UK charity providing Assistive Technology, and Augmentative and Alternative Communication services for people with complex needs. Ace Centre is based in Oldham and Abingdon, and the team offers assessment, training and information across England, including in areas with a sizable bilingual population.

In this chapter, the monolingual English-speaking team reflects on additional factors they consider when working with people who use AAC who understand and speak languages other than English.

## Introduction

Whilst many of the considerations when working with bilingual children raised in this book will also pertain to children who require Augmentative and Alternative Communication (AAC) resources to support their communication, there are additional factors that must be considered.

Despite the advantages of bilingualism for typically developing children being widely accepted and supported by the evidence base, there is often concern expressed by professionals and parents working with children with complex communication needs about providing communication supports in multiple languages (Yu, 2013). There is a common assumption that the learning of more than one language may be too difficult for those already experiencing challenges in their language learning, but this is not supported by the growing body of evidence in this area.

## László's story

László comes from a family where Hungarian, and English are spoken. He attends an English-speaking special needs school and has English-speaking carers at home for additional care at night times, weekends, and school holidays. When we first worked with László his family wished to focus on provision of AAC in English and said that it was not necessary to consider his Hungarian language needs as they had good English language skills. Eighteen months later his family got in touch to ask if we could now provide AAC in Hungarian. They had been pleasantly surprised by how well László had learnt to use AAC and how much he was now able to communicate. They now wanted him to have the opportunity to be able to communicate in Hungarian too. The family set-up had also changed as László's Grandparents, who do not speak English, moved into the family home. The main aim was now to give László access to the appropriate vocabulary on his AAC device so that he could join in games and socialise with his Grandparents.

The challenge for monolingual English-speaking professionals working with children who require AAC is that they often do not share a language with the service user they are supporting. It is important to find ways of working with service users in ways that support the development of language and interactions skills in the home language, regardless of whether that language is spoken by the professional.

## LANGUAGE AVAILABILITY AND NEED

### Equitable provision

When using a symbol based AAC system, an individual needs a complete, robust system that contains sufficient language to allow them to communicate all appropriate messages. The vocabulary included should reflect the way that a child or young person learns and how they use their language within their community. The vocabulary also needs to be culturally appropriate. It is essential to understand the underlying structure of the language a child is using, as consideration must be given to different modalities, vocabulary items, vocabulary designs and grammatical structures. This does not mean that every possible word in that language needs to be added. Instead, words are selected that cover a range of topics, including a high number of core words. Core words are words that are useful whatever the situation and to whoever you are speaking. For example, in English, these might be the pronouns "I," "you," "he," or "she"; verbs such as "go," "like," and "stop"; questions such as "who," "what," and "where"; or a range of other generic function words such as "more" and "not." These core words will differ depending on the semantic and syntactic structures of the home language.

When working with a bilingual or multilingual individual the ability to rapidly codeswitch between languages in the same utterance (intrasentential codeswitching) is also viewed as an authentic feature of bilingual communication. This will allow them to communicate in a similar way to a verbal bilingual speaker. Verbal speakers employ codeswitching for a variety of reasons, such as a means of expressing identity and solidarity within a social group, to select the most appropriate vocabulary item from any of their languages, or to signal an attitude towards a listener. This functions at a subconscious level for fluent verbal speakers. In contrast, due to the nature of electronic AAC, a bilingual speaker using AAC will always have to put a degree of conscious thought into codeswitching, as they navigate from one area of a programmed system to another. There are very few electronic AAC options that allow for page-by-page codeswitching between languages, and those that do exist still require a level of conscious thought to move between the languages.

## Jianyu's story

Jianyu is a seven-year-old boy who has autism. He attends a mainstream school where he is taught in English. His teachers and SLT agree that he understands English well, and he uses some English set phrases to communicate. At home, Jianyu's parents speak to him exclusively in Putonghua ("common language," also known as Mandarin). Neither of his parents speak English. Jianyu was provided with an AAC device to supplement his spoken communication. The vocabulary package selected was available in both English and Putonghua, listed as "Chinese (simplified)" on the supplier's website. Both language packages had been developed by native speakers, taking into account the different cultural considerations associated with each language. A bespoke solution was created by adding in links on every page to allow Jianyu to switch between the languages. This meant he was able to codeswitch when creating messages.

## Availability of AAC

There are few AAC resources available in languages other than English. There are more options for European languages such as French, Spanish, and German, but for many languages there are no ready-made options. Even for available languages, there are very few options that allow codeswitching. It may be that two languages can be used within one system, but if the navigation between the two is complex then it may impede the natural codeswitching that is frequently observed in spoken language.

Commercial AAC resources should always be evaluated for accuracy. A resource that has been made by a fluent speaker will more accurately represent the correct language constructs and word forms. In contrast, vocabularies which have been created using systems such as Google Translate should go through a rigorous evaluation process by a native speaker before being used, in order to ensure the translations are accurate and take into account the difference in underlying syntactic and semantic structures.

Due to the issues that can be encountered when identifying an AAC resource in a language other than English, it can be difficult to find a system that matches the requirements discussed above. If the SLT is not a native speaker of the language, a translator will be required to adapt the material. When creating a word-based symbol resource, this needs to be done in partnership with a professional who understands the purpose of the device and the language needs of the individual to ensure that translations are completed accurately. For example, consider the word "more." This is a core word commonly included in English AAC devices. It could also be translated as "additional," "extra," or "further." None of these translations are incorrect, but they do not accurately reflect the range of language functions that the word "more" covers in English. They also are less likely to be used by a child, so may not be appropriate to add to an AAC device.

Often a compromise must be found when creating a new AAC resource for a bilingual speaker. The time taken to create a full, robust system in a language other than English may mean an individual is left without any AAC until its completion. Instead, it may be that a smaller number of words and phrases are added to a device to start with, with further vocabulary added over time.

## Jolanta's story

Jolanta's mother is English, and her father is Polish. She has cerebral palsy and attends a mainstream high school. Jolanta uses AAC to augment her speech. Jolanta's family mainly speak English both at home and when out-and-about. However, her father identified certain topics/times of the day when he was more likely to speak in Polish with Jolanta and her siblings, such as conversations about household chores, leisure time and checking in with the children about their schoolwork. The English vocabulary package that Jolanta was using was not available in Polish and Jolanta was not literate in Polish. The compromise was that an alternative text-to-speech Polish vocabulary package was added to Jolanta's device with some pages of stored phrases that Jolanta and her siblings came up with. Jolanta had the skills to learn to use these phrases when she wanted to reply to her Dad in Polish – particularly to give her responses about doing chores and homework!

## Individual language needs

Different individuals will have different levels of second language need. Whilst some children may require fluency in two or more languages, others will benefit from a small number of words and phrases to allow them to participate in social conversations with their families and people in their communities.

## Alina's story

Alina is an eight-year-old girl who has cerebral palsy and is not able to use her spoken voice. Alina is from a British Pakistani community. Alina attends a special needs school where she uses her AAC device to share words and phrases in English to communicate with her friends and teachers. At home her family all speak English to each other, and Alina joins in by using her device.

Alina's family are Muslim, and in common with many families in the local community, her parents use Arabic and/or Urdu-Arabic religious phrases, especially for greetings. These include "As-salamu alaykum" ("Peace be upon you") used as a greeting, and when saying goodbye, "Khuda hafiz" ("God protect you"), although other variants are also common (see Ali, 2012). These phrases are fixed Islamic greetings which do not vary, and the family do not speak Arabic as a functional everyday language. Alina's parents use spoken Arabic blessings to each other and the children. Alina was keen to be able to join in with this practice, something that she has not been able to do before. Her Mum recorded the appropriate phrases onto a Step-by-Step digitised voice output device, which Alina then accessed using a single switch. Using this, Alina was able to greet her Dad when he returned home from work, and participate in sharing the spoken blessings.

## Words versus phrases

Most symbol based AAC systems contain a mixture of words and phrases. If a resource is being created from scratch, it is useful to consider the type of language that is usually contained in an AAC resource. As well as phrases for social interaction, the inclusion of words (particularly core words) alongside fringe (topic) vocabulary is useful as it allows an individual to generate novel utterances. It is important to include language that can be used in a range of settings, covering a range of pragmatic functions such as rejecting, requesting, commenting, and questioning.

Difficulties can arise when relying on family to generate the language – they are likely to focus on language that they feel will be useful, but this may not cover the wide range of language functions required by the child. For example, they may easily be able to generate phrases that will allow the child to participate in their daily routine (e.g., asking for help getting dressed, saying they need the toilet), but perhaps fail to consider language that the child might wish to use when playing with friends. A useful resource to support with the collection of language is the *Pragmatics Profile for People Who Use AAC* (Martin et al., 2017). This resource provides relevant interview questions to discuss an individual's use of language covering a range of pragmatic functions. It allows an in-depth look at each of these functions, and how well it is being communicated. This information can then be used to guide the development of an AAC resource that covers all of the relevant language functions.

A further consideration when translating single words is to ensure they are culturally appropriate. For example, the food options required in English may differ greatly to those required in Putonghua (Mandarin) or Polish, due to the cultural differences between the countries where these languages are spoken. Furthermore, the core words discussed above may differ between languages and cultures. The core words included in English-language systems have been generated following extensive research on English-speaking children. There may be minor differences in the core words of different languages, which should be considered when translating the material.

In English, the word "put" is often seen as a core word. You might say:

1.  "**Put** that down."
2.  "Where did you **put** it?"
3.  "**Put** your clothes on,"
4.  "**Put** my hair up."

However, in other languages such as Hindi, the semantic field covered by "put" in English is divided between different words, since the concept of "to put an object in a location" (utterances 1 and 2) are different than to "get dressed" and "arrange your hair" (utterances 3 and 4, respectively).

The work "rakh" is used in place of "put" for the first two options, where location is being encoded. Completely different words and utterance structures are used for phrases three and four. This demonstrates the error of assuming that direct translation of a set of core words will map onto a different language in the same way as English. Translation without cultural adaptation will not provide the same phrase structures and options as in the English language.

## Features

### Language specific voices

When using an electronic AAC device with voice output, there is a reliance on the availability of a synthesised voice in the relevant language to ensure that the messages are spoken out loud with the appropriate pronunciation (articulation and phonology). As each language is encoded using a different set of contrasting phonemes, pronunciation can be significantly affected by the use of a different voice. However, availability of synthesised voices is limited, particularly in languages other than English. It may be that only a male voice is available, or only a female voice, which does not match the gender of the service user. Similarly, the age of the voice may not match the service user, with only adult voices available. This means service users may only have the option of a voice that they do identify with.

In some instances, the phonemes and articulation of two languages may be similar enough that synthetic voices for the two languages may be used interchangeably. This is the case for Hindi and Urdu, which have very few differences in pronunciation. On some systems, only a Hindi voice can be used, and not an Urdu voice. However, as Hindi and Urdu are spoken in different countries and cultures, there are questions as to whether everyone would find it culturally appropriate to use a synthetic voice from the alternate language.

### Culturally appropriate symbols

Symbol systems are used by people who are unable to understand written text. Symbols are used on an AAC device to represent words and phrases, which are spoken out loud by the device when selected. An individual can combine these symbols to build messages to speak out loud, encompassing various levels of grammatical complexity.

Symbols are often used to represent language concepts. However, when selecting which symbols to use, clinicians are reliant on the bank of symbols which have been created previously. It may be that there are not symbols available for specific cultural practices, foods, or celebrations. In some of these situations, a generic symbol may be appropriate (for example, a "celebrate" or "party" symbol may be used to represent the Muslim festival of Eid), but there may be other situations where this not possible.

It is now much easier to find symbols covering a wider range of ethnicities and cultural practices, including, for example, symbols of a woman wearing a hijab or a man wearing a kippah. There are several producers of culturally appropriate symbol sets which can be appraised for their relevance to a specific individual (See Symbol Sets).

## ALLOCATING APPROPRIATE TIME TO ENSURE QUALITY OUTCOMES

### Time taken to create an AAC system

Off-the-shelf solutions for AAC, in particular, symbol-based systems, are developed over a period of months and years. These draw on expertise from several different individuals. When working with a monolingual English speaker, it is often possible to take an off-the-shelf solution and tweak it as needed to make it appropriate for a specific individual. However, when working with bilingual clients, this is not always possible. Although there is a growing number of resources available in languages other than English, this still covers a very small number of global languages. This means that resources must be created from scratch. This involves either translating and adapting a pre-existing resource or creating a bespoke resource containing words and phrases requested by the service user and their family. Both options take more time than working with an English monolingual service user to reach the same outcome: a usable AAC system which meets the needs of the service user. Therefore, double the time should be allocated to working with service users and their families from a bilingual community (Royal College of Speech and Language Therapists, 2022).

### Irtaza's story

Irtaza is a ten-year-old boy with diagnosed learning difficulties who attends a special needs school in England. Irtaza comes from a home where only Urdu is spoken. Irtaza is in and English-speaking classroom environment at school. Irtaza has a small amount of spoken language in English, but this is not representative of his level of verbal understanding across Urdu and English. He uses signs and symbols to support his communication but had previously only been given access to symbol resources in English. This meant he was unable to explore expression of Urdu at home without the provision of an additional solution. At present, there are no pre-set solutions available for electronic AAC in Urdu, meaning a bespoke solution was required to meet Irtaza's language needs in his home language.

We worked with Irtaza's Mum alongside a translator to collect a range of words and phrase she felt would be useful for him to use at home. These phrases were recorded and given to a transcriber who copied them into written Urdu. The phrases were then copied back on to the device. However, through these multiple steps, some errors were made meaning that the phrases had not been correctly entered into the device. Irtaza's parents are not literate in Urdu, so these mistakes could not be rectified. This identified a larger issue of how the device could be edited in the future.

After discussion with Dr Sean Pert, we used transliteration to enter the recorded phrases. This involved a broadly phonemic spelling of spoken Urdu using a Romanised keyboard. This was completed by a native Urdu speaker to improve accuracy of the transcription, as she was able to identify language-specific phonemes. These phrases were then spoken out loud using a male adult Hindi synthesised voice, as no Urdu synthesised voice was available. As Hindi and Urdu use the same phonemes, correct pronunciation of the phrases could be achieved. At present there is no commercially available male child synthesised voice for either Hindi or Urdu. This meant that the only choice was an adult male voice.

As there are no pre-set vocabularies available for Urdu, all language entered was selected by Irtaza's Mum. Although this meant he had access to words and phrases she felt were appropriate to him, it did not give access to as wide a range of vocabulary as is available in a pre-set system.

## ASSUMPTION OF LITERACY

## Text-to-speech systems

Text-to-speech systems are a common form of AAC used by people who are literate. Text is typed out on a keyboard, then spoken aloud by the device. This type of system provides many benefits for literate individuals, as it allows them to say precisely what they would like to, rather than selecting from a predetermined vocabulary set that has been defined by someone else. However, this type of system makes several assumptions:

1. The language being spoken has a standardised written form
2. This written form is alphabetical and easily transposed onto a keyboard
3. A relevant keyboard is available for the device
4. The individual using the system has a level of literacy that matches their verbal fluency.

The English alphabet has 26 letters. Many other modern languages have similar alphabets consisting of a relatively small number of characters, which are combined in various ways to form words. In contrast, scripted languages such as Putonghua (Mandarin) use characters to represent syllables and whole words alongside the alphabet, with a total of more than 70,000 whole-word characters used alongside the 33 graphemes making up the alphabet. This can make it extremely difficult to manage text entry on a device.

If an individual is exposed to more than one language, it is not uncommon that their language needs, including their need for literacy, will vary between the two. Someone may speak one language at home with family and friends, and an additional language at school (or other educational setting). They may have little reason to encounter the social language in its written form, and therefore have a level of literacy in the home language that is not representative of their understanding and potential use of the spoken language. Some languages have no written form, or access to education and literacy are limited.

Moreover, an individual may have had opportunity to learn how to physically write a language, but not to type it. This again presents difficulties when using a device which relies on the use of a keyboard.

The programming of a symbol-based system still requires a text-to-speech function to ensure the correct word or phrase is spoken when a symbol is selected. This makes the same assumptions of literacy discussed above, as a supporting adult will need to be able to enter written words in the appropriate language.

Consideration also needs to be given to cases where an individual has a physical disability which may lead to difficulty accessing an electronic AAC resource without support. For example, some individuals may benefit from having a keyguard to improve their ability to target areas of the screen. A keyguard is a plastic layer that is placed over the screen with holes that correspond to the keys on the screen, which helps to prevent the user from unintentionally pressing multiple keys. If we consider the example above of an individual who requires access to both the Putonghua (Mandarin) characters and English alphabet, difficulties may arise finding a keyguard which allows access to both of these language options simultaneously.

## Working with bilingual professionals

When working with an individual speaking a different language, an interpreter is required to ensure both parties can understand each other. In contrast, when it is written material that needs translating, a translator is employed. Problems can arise when working with

AAC as it may be that a combination of these two options is required, possibly alongside a transcription service to write down auditory information.

When collecting language for an AAC resource, this is often provided verbally by the family. This is either collected during an appointment or via audio recordings. This language sample is then transcribed to allow it to then be inputted into the device software, which then provides spoken output. Practical difficulties can arise when booking these services, as most services offer *either* interpreting *or* translation/transcription services separately, rather than as a combined option. This can mean having to work with several different services/individuals to reach the final product, which increases the opportunities for the introduction of errors at each stage.

## Meera's story

Meera's mother, Bhavna, was initially unsure about Meera's AAC device having Hindi content and mentioned that they could "make do without." It came to light that Bhavna's hesitancy was related to the fact that she found it effortful and time consuming to write in the Hindi script. We assured Bhavna that we could work with a translator to help add the Hindi content onto Meera's device and that we certainly did not want to make her responsible for another task on top of everything she already needed to do for her daughter's care. Bhavna was happy to audio-record the Hindi content for Meera's device and send us the files, as she could do this quickly and easily on her phone. There were challenges in finding the right professional to help us with the next steps. We booked an interpreter, but they did not agree to the job as there was no "live" interpretation happening. Similarly, a translator was not appropriate; Bhavna had supplied the English and the Hindi on the audio files, so as the agency pointed out there was no translation to be done! We learnt that a transcription service was required and found an agency that was happy to transcribe the audio files into a Word document. From there we could copy and paste the text into the AAC device. Unfortunately, this route meant that we were not working directly with a Hindi-speaking professional to help us trouble-shoot, and it meant that Bhavna had to take on the task of sense-checking the resource when it was handed over.

This illustrates that a native speaker who understands AAC would be best suited for tasks such as this - someone to whom the clinician can explain the work and who can input directly into the AAC software/vocabulary so that additional layers of work are not generated. This would be possible with a trained bilingual speech and language therapy assistant.

However, it isn't always possible to employ a home language speaker for each community, and so workarounds are required.

## CONSIDERATIONS FOR LONG-TERM IMPLEMENTATION OF AAC

### Ongoing support for personalisation

When a device is initially provided, it has often gone through a long stage of personalisation. Words and phrases relevant to the individual will have been added. This may include family names, favourite activities, and phrases that support social interaction in their relevant spheres. A translator or other native speaker may be involved at this stage to ensure that the phrases are entered correctly.

Once a device has been provided to an individual it is likely that further personalisation is required over time. The service user will use their AAC device more frequently and discover new activities and topics that they would like to discuss. This can cause issues if:

a.  there is not a literate adult in the family who can provide on-going support.
    That is, if family are fluent in the home language, but not *literate* in that language, and
b.  access to translation services is limited, as
    i.   the service user has been discharged from the speech and language therapy service, or
    ii.  there is not adequate instructional material to support navigation of the editing menu in the home language. Most systems are set up with the settings and edit mode in English. If a robust manual is not available in the home language, the family may not be able to carry out editing due to lack of language appropriate resources. This makes the assumptions of literacy in English, irrespective of their literacy in home language. Conversely, if an alternate language system is used – with all settings and menus also translated – this can cause difficulties for the professional supporting the individual.

On some occasions, spoken messages are recorded directly onto the device through a process referred to as "Message Banking." This negates the need for a synthesised voice and means an individual can access words or phrases with the correct pronunciation, tone, and intonation for any language. It is important to ensure that a plan is made for message banking in the future. If an interpreter is engaged to record the initial messages, it may be that their details are recorded for future bookings. If the phrases are recorded by a family member or friend, they should be informed of the expectation that they will be available for future recordings as well. An alternative plan should be agreed in the case of the designated individual being unavailable in the future.

## Language-specific therapy input

Much of AAC intervention focuses on the idea of modelling. That is, for an individual to be able to use a communication system effectively, they need to be shown how it works. This involves communication partners using the system alongside the learner, using the words and phrases in context to assign meaning to them. This AAC principle draws on pre-existing knowledge about the way that typical language learners acquire language.

Issues can arise if the learner does not have a skilled communication partner in all languages that they speak, as they will benefit from modelling in each language, rather than in only one. For example, they may have a skilled communication partner who only speaks English, with the home language only spoken with individuals who have not had access to training on how to model AAC. It is the responsibility of the professional to provide training to all relevant supporting adults in their own languages. This should be achieved with the help of an interpreter, preferably one who has experience and understanding of working with language development. Due to the subtleties of vocabulary structure and use in different languages, it is important to spend time with the interpreter discussing the strategies required to model the language appropriately.

It is important to consider the culturally appropriate interaction styles of a bilingual speaker, and the ways these may differ between the languages spoken. These interaction styles must form the basis of intervention plans in collaboration with the child's family.

## Things to consider when appraising an AAC resource in a language you do not share with the service user and their family

- **Who created the resource?**
  - Was it created by a native speaker?
  - Was it created by a linguist, Speech & Language Therapist or Pathologist, or generated by a translation process which does not consider cultural aspects? (Rather than adapted)

- **Is the resource available in your country?**

  If not, contact the company who make the resource and ask them to make it available. Sometimes the company haven't considered that the resource may be helpful to bilingual service users living in other countries.

- **Is the resource a translation of an English language AAC resource?**
  - Has the vocabulary been culturally adapted?
  - Have all aspects of the resource been translated?

  Sometimes the basic words and phrases have been translated but other features such as word prediction cells or operational function cells have not been.

- **Will the service user be able to easily move between this resource and an English AAC resource in order to code-switch?**

- **What text-to-speech voice options are there?**
  - Is there a voice available to go with the system?
  - Are there male voice and female voice options?
  - Are there adult voice and child voice options?
  - If there is no other choice than to use a text-to-speech voice that was created for a different language, consider how you will discuss this with the service user and their family. Be aware of any cultural sensitivities.

- **Is the resource available on a device that has the appropriate keyboard for the language available?**

  A keyboard matching the language will be essential for adding new words such as people's names and searching for words if there's a "search" function.

- **In which language are the settings/toolbox pages?**
  - Are there how-to guides available in English?
  - Will the clinician and others supporting the service user be able to learn how to use the system if they don't speak the language?

- **Can you work out how the language is organised in the resource?**
  - Does a cell trigger a single word or a whole phrase?
  - Is it possible to appraise the grammar options available?
  - Working with a native speaker of the language will be essential Find out if your local interpretation/translation service take bookings for this sort of work.

## Remember

Always be clear with a service user and their family when sharing an AAC resource that is in a language that you don't understand or speak. It won't be possible for you to have fully appraised the resource before they see it and as a consequence there may be inappropriate vocabulary or cultural insensitivities in the resource. Try to make sure the service user and their family feel empowered to tell you what is wrong with the resource!

## Symbol sets

https://globalsymbols.com/

https://arasaac.org/

https://globalsymbols.com/symbolsets/urdu-core-vocabulary-symbols

https://tawasol.mada.org.qa/main-symbol-page/

https://goboardmaker.com/

https://goboardmaker.com/blogs/news/additional-social-distancing-mask-and-diversity-symbols-pcs-update

www.widgit.com/about-symbols/widgit-symbols-2021/changes/people.htm

www.cricksoft.com/us/blog/crick/2021/02/03/symbolstix-diversity-update

## References

Ali, S. H. (2012, April 17). In Pakistan, saying goodbye can be a religious statement. *The Guardian*, Tuesday. Retrieved March 31, 2022, from www.theguardian.com/commentisfree/belief/2012/apr/17/pakistan-goodbye-allah-hafiz

Martin, S., Small, K. & Stevens, R. (2017). *The pragmatics profile for people who use AAC* (First Published 26 September 2017). Ace Centre. https://www.acecentre.org.uk/resources/pragmatics-profile-people-use-aac

Royal College of Speech and Language Therapists. (2022). *Clinical guidelines: Bilingualism guidance*. RCSLT. http://www.rcslt.org/members/clinical-guidance/bilingualism/bilingualism-guidance

Yu, B. (2013). Issues in bilingualism and heritage language maintenance: Perspectives of minority-language mothers of children with autism spectrum disorders. *American Journal of Speech-Language Pathology, 22*, 10-24. https://doi.org/10.1044/1058-0360(2012/10-0078)

# CULTURAL INQUISITIVENESS AND BILINGUAL SERVICE DELIVERY CHECKLIST

DOI: 10.4324/9781003125563-9

## Defining the problem

In both the US and UK, a lack of diversity is apparent in health care professions generally, with speech and language pathology/therapy being one of the least diverse health care professions (Guiberson & Vigil, 2021b; Moore et al., 2020).

Why does this matter, if the white cis heterosexual majority are dedicated professionals? There is evidence that ethnic, linguistic and socioeconomic (class) differences can interfere with access to, and the effective delivery of care, leading to poorer outcomes for service users and families from diverse backgrounds (Betancourt et al., 2003).

Failing to work alongside professional interpreters, especially with families who can "get by in English" (or the mainstream language), can lead to "malfunctioning encounters" with serious implications for misdiagnosis and treatment (Cambridge, 1999).

For families of bilingual children with developmental disabilities, SLTs fail to deliver services which follow professional guidelines and value home language(s). Marinova-Todd et al. (2016, p. 47) found that:

> "Regardless of clinical group, children who lived in homes where a minority language was spoken were often exposed to, assessed in, and treated in the majority language only; again, respondents (expert practitioners) generally disagreed with these practices"
>
> *(My brackets).*

Although ethnic diversity and bilingualism are not the same, many families will have intersectional identities. The high number of white monolingual SLTs has been associated with the maintenance of a predominantly mainstream English-only (or mainstream only) approach to assessment and intervention. This has been repeatedly reported in the literature for several decades, despite easy access to professional guidelines on home language in the US (ASHA) and the UK (RCSLT). This suggests one or more of the following:

- A negative attitude to languages other than the mainstream language such as English or Welsh
- Lack of cultural and linguistic awareness
- Ignorance of, or unwillingness to implement, professional guidelines, especially for children with disabilities or severe disorders
- Barriers such as cost of interpreters, lack of therapy time, lack of training opportunities, or attitudes of team leads and managers to home language approaches.

Both clinical and financial benefits have been associated with a great diversity in the workforce (Gomez & Bernet, 2019). These are powerful reasons for focusing on increasing diversity, as well as improving the individual experiences of Black, Asian, and ethnic families.

## Becoming an ally

Recruiting and educating allies who may not be diverse themselves is one way to improve the experiences of diverse individuals and families. As Case et al. (2020, p. 900) state, "potential allies hold the social power to question, challenge, and even redefine assumed norms that maintain oppression."

Many well-meaning professionals state that they are not racist personally, but then fail to be actively *anti-racist.* We live and work in institutions, including health provider organisations, which can be full of perfectly helpful, pleasant individuals, but the *system* or *care pathway* is intrinsically institutionally racist because, for example, bilingual families are given the same amount of time as monolingual English (mainstream language) speakers, ignoring the time taken to work alongside interpreters, plan culturally sensitive assessment, and discover information about the home language in order to plan intervention. Staffing may not reflect the communities served. Bilingualism may not be considered a clinical specialism. This state of affairs privileges white monolingual families not through active racism by individuals, but by failure to re-balance the system to address obvious disparities that require action, taking the perspective of families who may not be like you ("othering").

Changing this negative status quo is likely to mean challenging managers and team leads, highlighting professional clinical guidelines and having uncomfortable conversations about your own behaviours. Does it feel uncomfortable to challenge a manager when they state that interpreters are expensive and that you should "get by"? How much more uncomfortable it is for the families who cannot understand their child's needs or lose the ability to speak to their child in home language as they suffer language attrition. This has become a sensitive issue in the "culture war," where healthcare leaders have rejected the assertion by government bodies that institutional racism has finally been tackled (Lacobucci, 2021).

Allyship is not neutral and "performative allyship," where people in the privileged group declare that they are "not racist" or "not homophobic" personally, for example, and think that is sufficient. True allyship is part of life-long learning, and confronting your own privileges, which, if you are a cis white heterosexual person you may not even notice because you have never been subject to discrimination (see Thorne, 2022). Calling out discrimination even when people from the minority group are not there, challenging peers and taking the lead on uncomfortable conversations, and using professional and personal privilege and power to dismantle discrimination are important aspects.

Each individual's own life experience will make them more or less likely to identify with a particular community. Considering our personal reaction to LGBTQ+ people, disabled people, Black, Asian, and other ethnic people, those of a particular religion or belief, and so on is important work. We may be uncomfortable or find other ways of being alien to our own experience. Do you see people from these groups as equal partners, or patients to be pitied and helped? Full insight into our own reactions to "the other" is beyond the remit of this chapter and book. I do recommend that you explore these themes on an on-going basis and work with people from excluded or discriminated groups in a spirit of co-production.

## Increasing diversity in the workforce and representation

It is important that young people from all parts of the community are able to consider speech and language therapy as a career. In part, this is a vicious circle. The lack of role models from diverse backgrounds means that young people cannot always see themselves taking up this career path. Gabard (2007, p. 173) argues that "a critical mass of minorities within the student population plays a significant role in helping all students and practitioners to achieve cultural competency."

Engagement with young people through careers services, school engagement and via social media are important. There is bias in how the profession is represented. Byrne (2018, p. 426) conducted a study on how speech pathology services were portrayed online. Byrne concluded, "Images of speech pathology and professionals (speech pathologists) on the Internet are consistent with the current narrow professional demographic profile and it seems apparent that displaying that profile is only serving to continuing to perpetuate the lack of diversity as opposed to facilitating any change."

Recent changes demanded by Black, Asian, and ethnic members have led to more visual representation in professional magazines and web sites (Royal College of Speech and Language Therapists, 2020) following partnership with groups such as @SLTsofColour. This is part of a wider strategy and not merely a visual exercise. It is important not to focus solely on the presenting image of diversity if this is not followed up with substantial changes. This "optical allyship" is necessary but not sufficient to embed lasting change for people of colour (Thomas, 2018).

Guiberson and Vigil (2021a, p. 152) recommends consideration of "diversity assets" to improve recruitment, including "Bilingual/multilingual status, race/ethnicity, first-generation college educated, experience with disadvantage populations, gender, gender identity, gender presentation, identifying as lesbian, gay, bisexual, transgender or intersex, as well as socio-economic background."

## Intersectionality and LGBTQ+ people

"Culture" and "diversity" refer to more than just ethnicity. Gender, sexual orientation, and people with disability frequently face discrimination just for being who they are.

It is important to recognise that many people are members of more than one group which experiences discrimination. A person of colour may also be LGBTQ+ and experience homophobia, biphobia, or transphobia. That person may also experience discrimination both from within and outside of their community. A Black woman with a disability may experience misogyny and racism simultaneously. This is intersectionality, membership in two or more groups who experience discrimination, prejudice, stereotyping, and/or harassment.

The LGBTQ+ acronym refers to a person's sexual preference, romantic aims, and/or gender identity. These terms are *not concerned with sex*, but with *belonging* to a community. Lesbian, Gay, Bisexual, Trans(gender), and Queer people. The "+" denotes other identities and groups which form the community, which include people who are intersex, aromantic, asexual, and other identities. Terminology is evolving all the time to become more nuanced and respond to changes in society and the community. Please see Stonewall (2022). "Trans" is an abbreviation of "transgender," which is itself an umbrella term covering a range of gender identities including non-binary people. Please see LGBT Foundation (2022).

In the UK, almost one in eight LGBT people have experienced some form of unequal treatment from healthcare staff because they're LGBT, and almost one in four have witnessed discriminatory or negative remarks against LGBT people by healthcare staff (Bachmann & Gooch, 2018). Similarly, in the US LGBTQ+ people face discrimination from healthcare providers, with reports of "multiple examples of microaggressions and healthcare provider discomfort" (Smith & Turell, 2017).

LGBTQ+ people may be parent(s) to a child with a speech, language, or communication disorder and/or developmental disability. The assumption that all parent(s)/carers and children and young people are cis gendered (identify as the same gender they were assigned at birth) and heterosexual is known as *cisheteronormativity*. This also impacts on students on clinical placement in speech and language therapy services and staff working in these services.

Individual practitioners and services should evaluate their paperwork, questions and assessment and therapy materials to ensure that LGBTQ+ people are made to feel welcome and that assumptions are not made about their gender and sexual identity. Visible allyship such as Rainbow Flag/Progress Flag lanyards, display boards and posters featuring LGBTQ+ people, and including Black, Asian, and LGBTQ+ people with a wide variety of different ethnicities are powerful ways of making the environment friendly to staff and service users alike.

Speech and language therapists have a potential role with transgender children and youth who may wish to change their voice and communication (Hancock & Helenius, 2012). Some of these children will be bilingual and/or from a cultural background that is not the same as the mainstream.

When changing gender identity, cultural identity may become important in the way that they interpret their transgender status. Many cultures prior to contact with white western society accepted individuals who rejected the gender binary or identified with a gender not assigned at birth. Examples include the Hijra of the Indian sub-continent (Newport, 2018); Māhū of Hawaii, Tahiti and Bora Bora (Besnier & Alexeyeff, 2014); and the fa'afafine of Polynesia. Such identities were often not stigmatised by these cultures, and it is the western pathologising medical model view of gender difference which led to the characterisation of gender diversity as a mental disorder. Research into individuals from these cultures who are often more tolerant of gender variance may help western society to re-evaluate this medicalisation. Vasey and Bartlett (2007, p. 489) in their study of fa'afafine individuals found that "there is no sound evidence that cross-gender behaviors or identities, per se, cause distress."

Speech and language therapists working with trans people of colour should receive additional training to support their work with Trans People of Colour (TPOC) communities (Choudrey, 2022).

## Intersectionality and people with a disability

People with disabilities face discrimination, harassment, and antisocial behaviour directed at them simply because they have a disability. With large numbers of cases of harassment of people with disabilities, and many more unreported, "Disabled people are expected to be flexible and adapt, to fit into the hostile world rather than the society changing." (Capewell et al., 2015, p. 217).

Shaw et al. (2012, p. 88) noted that in the US "various combinations of specific characteristics, that is, being female, being older, having a behavioral disability, racial minority status … seem to place individuals at higher risk of experiencing disability harassment."

Similarly, LGBT+ people with a disability are subject to higher levels of discrimination. Toft and Franklin (2020, p. 6) noted "astonishing levels of discrimination based on the triad of minority statuses: being young, being LBGT+ and being disabled."

As speech and language therapists we must, therefore, ensure that our practice and services are welcome to all, with efforts to ensure that children and young people with a range of diverse characteristics are included and their needs recognised.

## Socioeconomic status (social class)

Different socioeconomic background, or social class, can act as a barrier to effective healthcare (Guiberson & Vigil, 2021b). Healthcare providers, including speech and language therapists may assume that families are able to understand technical terminology, read to a proficient level, have access to toys, drawing and other play materials, and have the same interaction style and free time to provide therapy at home.

Assumptions that parent(s) and carers can read to a high level is particularly pervasive in speech and language therapy. Often, parent(s) and carers are provided with information on their child's diagnosis, or an intervention in the form of a written information leaflet. Such information may be difficult to read and include difficult words (Pothier et al., 2008).

Parents' interaction styles tend to vary with socioeconomic status (SES), with education and income, with *on average* parents with more years of education and income likely to use more words, longer utterances and less directive styles of interaction with young children. There are, of course, individual differences. Rowe (2018, p. 124) reported that "Parents with more education may be more likely than parents with less education to turn to health professionals or written materials for information about parenting."

## Student education

The teaching of bilingualism and cultural diversity should be incorporated into the curriculum of speech and language therapy/pathology pre-qualification programmes. Many universities teach topics such as child language development, and speech sound development, and their associated disorders as if they are restricted to monolingual children speaking a high-status language, mainly English. This bias leads to the assumption that any child who does not follow observed stages, patterns, or order of acquisition, or does not conform to "normal limits" on normative data, are in some way disordered and therefore merit treatment. The reliance on standardised assessments and normative data based on monolingual populations simplifies clinical decisions to the point where the holistic identity of the child or young person may be lost.

Despite evidence from hundreds of language communities across the globe, there is still an assumption that bilingualism has a negative impact on children's speech and language development. I am aware of no study that has ever implicated bilingualism in a speech or language disorder. Having two or more languages certainly means a *different* experience of speech and language acquisition, but the personal, social and employment benefits of bilingualism certainly outweigh any short-term cost of needing more time than a monolingual child to acquire the mainstream language.

Similarly, awareness of other cultures, including child-rearing, play, parent-child interaction and other heavily culturally-influenced traditions should also be taught. Too often, deviation from a western middle-class pattern of child rearing and interaction is seen as aberrant and unacceptable. Instead of valuing equally appropriate ways of raising children, too often professionals chide parents and carers from other cultures for their non-conforming, or worse "uneducated" or "ill-informed," style of parenting.

One example is parent-child interaction therapy (PCIT) for Language Difficulties in young children. A widely used (Falkus et al., 2016), valid, and appropriate approach, PCIT was developed with middle-class white parents, encouraging them to follow the child's lead. Awde, (2009, p. 14) found that "in many Asian minority communities, directing the child's lead, attention directing and teaching explicitly prevail, meaning that therapist's recommendations can interfere with the family dynamics and may encourage parents to interrupt therapy." This matches my clinical experience where bilingual parents from Pakistani- and Bangladeshi-heritage families have found direct language groups, where the speech and language therapist works directly with their child, more acceptable than a PCIT group.

Such adaptations, taking into account the needs of a particular community, their culture, and their own experiences, are part of evidence-based practice (EBP) (Klatte & Roulstone, 2016). This aspect, of adapting and including the unique perspective of families, is often forgotten in the application of EBP. Teaching students examples of selecting interventions that match and value a family's interaction style would be helpful in avoiding a "one size fits all" approach, often leading to poor outcomes and families disengaging from therapy.

In Speech Sound Disorder (SSD), it has been found that intervention in one language for a Phonological Delay or Consistent Phonological Disorder does not generalise to the other language(s), and that bilingual children "had language-specific phonological systems" (Holm et al., 1997). The underlying disorder was the same, with error patterns addressed in that particular language. This means that if therapy is delivered in only English, the child's difficulties in home language (Punjabi) would persist. If students were taught phonology from a bilingual perspective, then the importance of conceptualising the phonological system as the interface between the lexicon/language and the speech encoding system (rather than articulation, the physical production of phones using the vocal tract) becomes highly relevant. Intervention in English would *obviously* not interact with the home language, as they are entirely different phonological (contrastive) systems. This is but one example where utilising bilingual case studies to teach speech and language acquisition and disorders would clarify, not complicate pedagogy and encourage future practitioners to value their bilingual service users.

Case-based learning should include diverse families so that students can learn to balance professional sensitivity, cultural awareness, and the need to discover information about a family. For example, LGBT+ parents, bilingual parents, or those with disabilities could be the parent of a case study on a child with language disorder. This helps the theme of diversity break out of a silo of "Bilingualism" or "Multiculturalism" which may be ignored or avoided, especially if provided as an optional unit.

Including topics such as "Working with Interpreters" under an umbrella of "Multi-disciplinary Team Working" (MDT) will embed bilingualism into professional practice learning. If interpreters are seen as a key member of the MDT, alongside paediatricians, geneticists, teachers, health visitors, and other professionals, then the message that they are integral, rather than peripheral, to the MDT is given.

## Improving services by harnessing community power: Co-production

While services continue to be unrepresentative of the communities that they serve, professionals cannot hope to perceive service delivery from the perspective of diverse service users and families. By definition, professionals are highly educated and earn significantly more than many of the families they meet in clinician practice. So, how can we identify the barriers to accessing and engaging with services?

Co-production is "a collaborative process in which key stakeholders . . . work(ed) together in a structured and facilitated way" (Wray et al., 2021, p. 4, my brackets). Co-production in speech and language therapy services has been reported in relation to stroke survivors with aphasia, and trans and gender diverse people undergoing voice and communication change (Pert et al., 2021).

Marshall et al. (2017, p. 497) sought the views of parents that speech and language therapy managers in England considered under-served. Parents interviewed included carers of looked after children, minority ethnic groups, and those with low socio-economic status. They "wanted professionals to take time to get to know them, their child and their context in a non-judgemental way before making judgments."

Involving bilingual families to help design and evaluate your service can help to ensure that it is welcoming and fit for purpose. Examples include:

- Appointing a service user group to advise the service*
- Asking bilingual families to review your service*

- Collecting service evaluation questionnaires**
- Conducting service user interviews on their experiences*
- Publishing "you said, we did" posters and newsletters in languages spoken in your local area
- Undertaking quality checklists (see below).

*With the involvement of an interpreter; **For those families who are literate.

The advantage of the co-production model is that services can avoid problems and mistakes before they arise. Complaints can be seen as opportunities to improve the service, and actively seeking feedback can elicit compliments as well as suggestions.

## Cultural inquisitiveness

Many people talk of "cultural competence" in relation to speech and language clinical practice (Guiberson & Vigil, 2021b; Leadbeater & Litosseliti, 2014).

In discussion with bilingual speech and language therapists, RCSLT adopted "cultural inquisitiveness" to highlight that one is never really completely fully able to understand a culture one does not share or participate in. Rather, an open-minded attitude, where the person or family from that community is seen as the expert, allows the profession to work in partnership to deliver assessment, therapy, and advice which is sensitive to the family's culture and perspective.

The following is a checklist for individual professionals or services, which includes a section on cultural inquisitiveness.

## RCSLT checklist: essential Foundations for working successfully with bilingual children experiencing SLCN and their families

The following is *adapted* from the Royal College of Speech and Language Therapists' checklist developed to support students, practitioners and services to consider how their practice meets the clinical guidelines on working with bilingual children and their families (Pert & Shah, 2021).

*All* the following essential steps apply to *all* bilingual clients regardless of age group, except where "child" is specifically stated (and even for these steps, the principle still applies).

| *Pre-referral and referral* | | *Progress/status* | | |
|---|---|---|---|---|
| *Essential step* | *Evidence and RCSLT Guidance* | *Achieved* | *Working towards* | *Not evidenced* |
| 1. The **languages and dialects spoken** in the local area are **listed on the referral form.** The list is based on published statistics. | Generic terms such as "Chinese" instead of a specific language, such as "Cantonese," or "Pakistani" instead of "Urdu," should alert the SLTs that the referring agent is either unfamiliar with the local community's languages or has not sufficiently checked the family language. High-status languages are often reported, when the family may speak a related but less well-known language. | | | |
| 2. A **three-way telephone or video conference call is arranged** with the client/family, **interpreter** and speech and language therapist in order to check the client's language(s) and to answer any questions about the appointment. | Correct identification of the child and family's language(s) is crucial to ensuring good relationships with the family and reaching any diagnostic decisions. Telephone triage is therefore an essential component of working with bilingual families prior to booking face-to-face interpreters. | | | |
| 3. **An interpreter is booked prior to the session** to review assessment/ intervention materials, discuss cultural appropriateness and plan translation and adaptation of materials. **Only professional interpreters over 18 are acceptable. Family members under 18 should never be asked to fulfil this role.** | The interpreter and SLTs should work together to identify any cultural or linguistic issues which may arise. Collaborating with professional interpreters should not be viewed as optional and must not be restricted by budgetary constraints. | | | |
| 4. **The appointment format is accessible for the client/family.** This may include a letter in the majority language (such as English or Welsh) with a QR code to an audio version in home language. | Websites including verbal as well as written translations of referral information and help and advice The use of text-based translation, text-to-speech and speech-to-text translation, and other machine-based translation | | | |

| Pre-referral and referral | | Progress/status | | |
| --- | --- | --- | --- | --- |
| *Essential step* | *Evidence and RCSLT Guidance* | *Achieved* | *Working towards* | *Not evidenced* |
| Note that many clients/ families cannot read their home language, check at the three-way appointment.<br>Translating letters and leaflets into home language scripts may be less useful than verbal translations for many communities.<br>Do not use computer text translation. | rely on non-human algorithms. Although such translation systems are improving at rapid rates and are readily accessible on personal computers and mobile devices, they cannot currently provide an acceptable alternative to human interpreters.<br>Other pitfalls include the possible transmission of Patient Identifiable Data across the internet in an unencrypted form, processing outside the UK or outside the European Union and other data transmission, as well as processing and storage – which may be hidden from the user.<br>The use of IT-based translation systems are therefore highly likely to compromise confidentiality and Information Governance legislation, including the Data Protection Act (1998) and the General Data Protection Regulation (Data Protection Act 2018, 2022). | | | |
| **Assessment and intervention** | | | | |
| 5.  Each contact with a client should include the following, in partnership with an interpreter:<br>• **Planning time**<br>• **The session**<br>• **A debrief** to discuss the session outcomes and any cultural and translation queries arising<br>• **Double the time allocated** for a typical monolingual client should be allowed for adaptations and the translation process (equitable service). | Services should allocate at least double the time at all stages, including assessment and intervention for bilingual clients and their families, in order to achieve the same positive outcomes as monolingual clients. | | | |

(*Continued*)

| | Pre-referral and referral | | Progress/status | | |
| --- | --- | --- | --- | --- | --- |
| | *Essential step* | *Evidence and RCSLT Guidance* | *Achieved* | *Working towards* | *Not evidenced* |
| 6. | If the client only has difficulty working in the majority language/ language of education (such as English, Welsh or Gaelic), then the client has an additional language need, and this is *not* the role of the speech and language therapist. Such clients should be referred to specialist teaching staff. | If there is a communication disorder, then it will be present in both/all the languages that the individual understands and uses. | | | |
| 7. | The **care plan will be delivered in home language** and/or both languages. **Home language aims will be achieved** prior to delivering the programme in English/ language of education. Speech and language therapists should recommend a **home language approach** in the care plan and report recommendations. | A written care plan should be written in collaboration with the parent(s)/carer specifying the speech and/or language therapy aims. This should specify the language in which the therapy will be provided, and that the child must be successful in their home language prior to attempting the same targets in their additional language. Ideally the staff expected to provide support should be agreed and named and resources identified, along with the "dose" (number of minutes per session and number of sessions per week). This should be **double the time** than when working with a monolingual English-speaking child. The aims should be outcomes focused and the treatment intensity merely a guide to minimum input. The agreed support is important as the amount of input is crucial to maintaining success. | | | |
| 8. | The **parent/carer interview** (case history) must include a **language exposure and usage interview**. | Attitudes to the home language and the language of education should be discussed. Parents may have absorbed myths about bilingualism or feel that education in the majority language is more important than maintaining | | | |

| Pre-referral and referral | | Progress/status | | |
|---|---|---|---|---|
| *Essential step* | *Evidence and RCSLT Guidance* | *Achieved* | *Working towards* | *Not evidenced* |
| | home language, without considering the negative impacts on the child and the family.<br><br>The first interview with a bilingual adult or family member/carer is crucial to establish rapport and gather functionality aspects of the use of the mother tongue (L1) and exposure to the mainstream/majority language (L2), or any other languages used. | | | |
| 9. | **Assessment is carried out in home language** if a child has yet to develop the majority language or in both/all languages if they have started to acquire two or more languages.<br><br>This applies to speech development as well as language development since bilingual children may have different surface errors in each of their languages, and intervention for phonological errors does not generalise from one language to another. | Assessing both/all languages to determine whether a language learning difficulty exists, to capture skills in both languages and to assess code-switching – which is likely to provide the longest and most representative language samples (Pert & Letts, 2006). This requires bilingual-to-bilingual communication and so an interpreter is essential for language assessment. | | |
| 10. | For **assessment of** speech or language, **home language should be recorded if used by the client, not just the translation.**<br><br>A translation protocol should be used. | Translation grids are used in order to preserve the child's original utterance and to make the stages of translation transparent. | | |
| 11. | **Published assessments should be adapted,** *never* **translated.**<br><br>If published assessments are used, standard scores must not be used for diagnosis, nor quoted on reports, nor used as criteria for access to specialist provision. | With such huge differences between monolingual children and bilingual, bi-cultural children, in terms of language exposure and cultural experience, SLTs must not quote:<br>• age equivalents<br>• standard scores<br>• percentile ranks; or | | |

(*Continued*)

| | Pre-referral and referral | | Progress/status | | |
|---|---|---|---|---|---|
| | *Essential step* | *Evidence and RCSLT Guidance* | *Achieved* | *Working towards* | *Not evidenced* |
| | Informal, culturally appropriate assessment materials are superior to direct translations of published assessments in English. | • other similar normative data derived from monolingual English-speaking populations. | | | |
| 12. | **Intervention aims should be achieved in home language** and then in English. | There is high-risk of home language loss for bilingual children who are treated in English (or the language of education), rather than their home language. The risk increases for low-status language speakers. Language loss is rapid, occurring in a few months and is often irreversible. SLTs should therefore offer home language intervention, prior to therapy in the language of education (English, Gaelic, or Welsh), especially for sequential bilinguals. | | | |

**Cultural inquisitiveness: language, cultural practices, and religion**

| | | | | | |
|---|---|---|---|---|---|
| 13. | The speech and language therapist will have an attitude of **cultural inquisitiveness**, also known as cultural competence development. Remember that you will *not* achieve some mythical level of cultural competence; this is an on-going process. SLTs will utilise their **reflective log** to monitor their development in the areas of languages, culture and religion. Language transmits culture and helps individuals to access support from their family, extended family and wider community. Home language and/or additional languages may be employed to | It is the responsibility of the SLT to become culturally competent by having an ongoing awareness of how their own cultural biases may affect the service. In other words, the process of cultural competence originates with each of us – we all have our own culture which will impact on practice. | | | |

| Pre-referral and referral | | Progress/status | | |
| --- | --- | --- | --- | --- |
| *Essential step* | *Evidence and RCSLT Guidance* | *Achieved* | *Working towards* | *Not evidenced* |
| access the client and family's religion. SLTs should **educate themselves** about the cultural practises, beliefs, religion and languages used by their clients, without expecting all families within a community to have the same expression of these aspects (stereotyping). This should be part of your ongoing CPD. **SLTs should include questions on language use, cultural practices, beliefs and religion. These questions should be asked in a respectful manner and not include superfluous information. Explain why you need information from clients** and how this will be used to **understand their needs and plan their care.** **Clients should not be expected to educate professionals** on their language, culture, beliefs and religion. | | | | |
| 14. | **Culturally appropriate resources** should be used in discussion with the interpreter/adult informant. | The interpreter and SLTs should work together to identify any cultural or linguistic issues which may arise. | | |

**Outcome**

| | | | | |
| --- | --- | --- | --- | --- |
| 15. | Overall **outcome should be that the client maintains/develops home language** alongside the language of education/majority language. | The main aim of intervention with bilingual clients is to maintain, restore or achieve bilingualism. | | |

**Further learning, allyship and supporting colleagues**

| | | | | |
| --- | --- | --- | --- | --- |
| 16. | **SLTs should see learning about other languages, cultural practice, beliefs, and religion as a life-** | See Strategies to increase cultural competency: www.rcslt.org/-/media/Project/RCSLT/8-strat-increase-cult-comp.pdf | | |

*(Continued)*

| | Pre-referral and referral | | Progress/status | | |
|---|---|---|---|---|---|
| | Essential step | Evidence and RCSLT Guidance | Achieved | Working towards | Not evidenced |
| | **long process.** It is acceptable to have an attitude of respect for others' way of life, but have limited knowledge, as long as you are committed to discovering more. | | | | |
| 17. | The profession in the UK is composed of a majority of white monolingual English-speaking SLTs. It is important that this more privileged section of the SLT community supports those from bilingual and/or those from Black, Asian, and minority ethnic backgrounds and those with diverse heritage.<br>This should involve:<br>• **actively challenging racism** in the workplace<br>• **undertaking training and CPD** on bilingualism, cultures different to your own, and on religion<br>• **becoming aware of your own culture, beliefs** and how they might influence your own practice<br>• **encouraging colleagues to do the same** | See cultural competence checklist: www.rcslt.org/-/media/ Project/RCSLT/9-cult-competence-checklist.pdf | | | |

| Signature of supervisor/mentor: | Date: |
|---|---|
| | |

## Sign off

Please ensure that your clinical supervisor or mentor signs off the above following implementation and discussion. Remember, learning is not completed until applied to a service user and you have reflected on that implementation.

## Next steps

This is not a comprehensive check list.

Please work as a team to improve the service in order to be equitable to all clients. This includes:

- carrying out CPD
- reading and applying RCSLT clinical guidelines
- accessing training courses
- joining a Clinical Excellence Network (CEN)
- carrying out/contributing to audits to ensure best practice is applied throughout the service by all staff

Bilingual staff and those from diverse communities should not necessarily lead on service change and development. Students and speech and language therapists with *any* level of home language skill are encouraged to use these skills to make clients feel welcome, even if working alongside a required interpreter. It is the responsibility of all speech and language therapists to value bilingualism and cultural diversity and to actively challenge racism. This applies to both our clients and our colleagues.

## To reference this checklist

Pert, S. & Shah, S. (2021). *Essential foundations for working successfully with bilingual children experiencing SLCN and their families*. Royal College of Speech and Language Therapists. www.rcslt.org

## References

Bachmann, C. L., & Gooch, B. (2018). *LGBT in Britain: Health report*. Stonewall. http://www.stonewall.org.uk/system/files/lgbt_in_britain_health.pdf

Besnier, N., & Alexeyeff, K. (Eds.). (2014). *Gender on the edge: Transgender, gay and other Pacific Islanders*. University of Hawai'i Press.

Betancourt, J. R., Green, A. R., Carrillo, J. E., & Ananeh-Firempong Ii, O. (2003). Defining cultural competence: A practical framework for addressing racial/ethnic disparities in health and health care. *Public Health Reports (1974)*, *118*, 293–302. https://doi.org/10.1016/S0033-3549(04)50253-4

Byrne, N. (2018). Internet images of the speech pathology profession. *Australian Health Review*, *42*, 420–428. https://doi.org/10.1071/AH17033

Cambridge, J. (1999). Information loss in bilingual medical interviews through an untrained interpreter. *The Translator*, *5*, 201–219. https://doi.org/10.1080/13556509.1999.10799041

Capewell, C., Ralph, S., & Bonnett, L. (2015). The continuing violence towards disabled people. *Journal of Research in Special Educational Needs*, *15*, 211–221. https://doi.org/10.1111/1471-3802.12112

Case, K. A., Rios, D., Lucas, A., Braun, K., & Enriquez, C. (2020). Intersectional patterns of prejudice confrontation by White, heterosexual, and cisgender allies. *Journal of Social Issues*, *76*, 899–920. https://doi.org/10.1111/josi.12408

Choudrey, S. (2022). *Supporting trans people of colour.* Jessica Kingsley.

Data Protection Act 2018. (2022). Retrieved August 10, 2022, from https://www.legislation.gov.uk/ukpga/2018/12/contents/enacted

Falkus, G., Tilley, C., Thomas, C., Hockey, H., Kennedy, A., Arnold, T., . . . Pring, T. (2016). Assessing the effectiveness of parent – child interaction therapy with language delayed children: A clinical investigation. *Child Language Teaching & Therapy, 32,* 7–17. https://doi.org/10.1177/0265659015574918

Gabard, D. L. (2007). Increasing minority representation in the health care professions. *Journal of Allied Health, 36,* 165–175.

Gomez, L. E., & Bernet, P. (2019). Diversity improves performance and outcomes. *Journal of the National Medical Association, 111,* 383–392. https://doi.org/10.1016/j.jnma.2019.01.006

Guiberson, M., & Vigil, D. C. (2021a). Speech-language pathology graduate admissions: Implications to diversify the workforce. *Communication Disorders Quarterly, 42,* 145–155. https://doi.org/10.1177/1525740120961049

Guiberson, M., & Vigil, D. C. (2021b). Admissions type and cultural competency in graduate speech-language pathology curricula: A national survey study. *American Journal of Speech-Language Pathology, 30,* 2017–2027. https://doi.org/10.1044/2021_AJSLP-20-00324

Hancock, A., & Helenius, L. (2012). Adolescent male-to-female transgender voice and communication therapy. *Journal of Communication Disorders, 45,* 313–324. https://doi.org/10.1016/j.jcomdis.2012.06.008

Holm, A., Dodd, B., Stow, C., & Pert, S. (1997). Speech disorder in bilingual children: Four case studies. *Osmania Papers in Linguistics, 22-23,* 45–64.

Klatte, I. S., & Roulstone, S. (2016). The practical side of working with parent- child interaction therapy with preschool children with language impairments. *Child Language Teaching and Therapy, 32,* 345–359. https://doi.org/10.1177/0265659016641999

Lacobucci, G. (2021). Healthcare leaders reject "damaging" denial that institutional racism exists. *BMJ (Online), 373,* n911. https://doi.org/10.1136/bmj.n911

Leadbeater, C., & Litosseliti, L. (2014). The importance of cultural competence for speech and language therapists. *Journal of Interactional Research in Communication Disorders, 5*(1), 1–26. https://doi.org/10.1558/jircd.v5i1.1

LGBT Foundation. (2022). *The basics.* LGBT Foundation. https://www.lgbt.foundation/smirnoff/the-basics

Marinova-Todd, S. H., Colozzo, P., Mirenda, P., Stahl, H., Kay-Raining Bird, E., Parkington, K., . . . Genesee, F. (2016). Professional practices and opinions about services available to bilingual children with developmental disabilities: An international study. *Journal of Communication Disorders, 63,* 47–62. https://doi.org/10.1016/j.jcomdis.2016.05.004

Marshall, J., Harding, S., & Roulstone, S. (2017). Language development, delay and intervention-the views of parents from communities that speech and language therapy managers in England consider to be under-served. *International Journal of Language & Communication Disorders, 52,* 489–500. https://doi.org/10.1111/1460-6984.12288

Moore, I., Bitchell, L., & Lord, R. (2020). *The health & care professions council equality, diversity and inclusion data 2020 report.* Health & Care Professions Council. www.hcpc-uk.org/globalassets/about-us/edi/hcpc-equality-diversity-and-inclusion-data-2020-report.pdf?v=637395820190000000

Newport, S. (2018). *Writing otherness: Uses of history and mythology in constructing literary representations of India's hijras.* University of Manchester. www.research.manchester.ac.uk/portal/en/theses/writing-otherness-uses-of-history-and-mythology-in-constructing-literary-representations-of-indias-hijras(d884b37f-417b-478d-9f19-e00d2129c327).html

Pert, S., Cheng, N., & Jenner, L. (2021, October 5–7) Published. *Online voice and communication change groups for trans and non-binary people.* Royal College of Speech and Language Therapists' Conference 2021: Breaking barriers and building better. www.research.manchester.ac.uk/portal/en/publications/online-voice-and-communication-change-groups-for-trans-and-nonbinary-people(6c53f987-28d2-449d-b629-b4c624b2f661).html

Pert, S., & Letts, C. (2006). Codeswitching in Mirpuri speaking Pakistani heritage preschool children: Bilingual language acquisition. *The International Journal of Bilingualism: Cross-disciplinary, Cross-linguistic Studies of Language Behavior, 10*(3), 349–374. https://doi.org/https://doi.org/10.1177/13670069060100030501

Pert, S., & Shah, S. (2021). *Essential foundations for working successfully with bilingual children experiencing SLCN and their families.* Royal College of Speech and Language Therapists. www.rcslt.org

Pothier, L., Day, R., Harris, C., & Pothier, D. D. (2008). Readability statistics of patient information leaflets in a Speech and Language Therapy Department. *International Journal of Language & Communication Disorders, 43*(6), 712–722. https://doi.org/10.1080/13682820701726647

Rowe, M. L. (2018). Understanding socioeconomic differences in parents' speech to children. *Child Development Perspectives, 12,* 122–127. https://doi.org/10.1111/cdep.12271

Royal College of Speech and Language Therapists. (2020). *Black lives matter: An update on the RCSLT's diversity and anti-racism work. 24th July 2020.* RCSLT. www.rcslt.org/news/rcslt-update-on-anti-racism-and-diversity-work

Shaw, L. R., Chan, F., & McMahon, B. T. (2012). Intersectionality and disability harassment: The interactive effects of disability, race, age, and gender. *Rehabilitation Counseling Bulletin, 55,* 82–91. https://doi.org/10.1177/0034355211431167

Smith, S. K., & Turell, S. C. (2017). Perceptions of healthcare experiences: Relational and communicative competencies to improve care for LGBT people: LGBT healthcare experiences. *Journal of Social Issues, 73,* 637–657. https://doi.org/10.1111/josi.12235

Stonewall. (2022). *List of LGBTQ+ terms.* Stonewall. www.stonewall.org.uk/help-advice/faqs-and-glossary/list-lgbtq-terms

Thomas, L. (2018, May 1). We are not interested in optical allyship. *Instagram.* Retrieved March 9, 2022, from www.instagram.com/p/BiPDZkbFJFY/?hl=en

Thorne, S. (2022). Moving beyond performative allyship. *Nursing Inquiry, 29,* e12483. https://doi.org/10.1111/nin.12483

Toft, A., & Franklin, A. (2020). Sexuality and gender identity in the lives of young, disabled LGBT+ persons. In A. Franklin & A. Toft (Eds.), *Young, disabled and LGBT+: Voices, identities and intersections.* Routledge.

Vasey, P. L., & Bartlett, N. H. (2007). What can the Samoan "fa'afafine" teach us about the western concept of gender identity disorder in childhood? *Perspectives in Biology and Medicine, 50,* 481–490. https://doi.org/10.1353/pbm.2007.0056

Wray, F., Clarke, D., Cruice, M., & Forster, A. (2021). Development of a self-management intervention for stroke survivors with aphasia using co-production and behaviour change theory: An outline of methods and processes. *PLoS One, 16,* e0259103. https://doi.org/10.1371/journal.pone.0259103

# BARRIERS TO WORKING WITH BILINGUAL CHILDREN AND HOW TO OVERCOME THEM

### CAROL STOW

DOI: 10.4324/9781003125563-10

# Barriers to working with bilingual children and how to overcome them

The need to provide an equitable service to bilingual children is enshrined in various laws and in professional guidelines. This book has outlined both the theoretical issues and the practical solutions which need to be considered when offering such a service. Despite this, many bilingual families will encounter barriers which are erected by SLTs and which prevent an equitable service from being offered. Below, these barriers are considered as frequently encountered statements with the solutions provided.

## I'm not allowed the additional time needed

It is the role of the SLT to advocate for the needs of their local community. Without knowledge of the demographics of the local bilingual communities, it is not possible to gauge if they are providing a service which meets the needs of this local bilingual population.

Audit is a powerful and persuasive tool. Team leads, service managers and commissioners of services will find it difficult to ignore statistics. SLTs should therefore be pro-active in submitting reports which contain statistical data describing the current service offering in relation to local bilingual populations and contrast this with the service offered to local monolingual, majority language speaking children and their families. Several factors need to be considered when developing such reports:

- Consider that the age profile of your local population may be different from the overall population. A community with a younger demographic profile will have a greater need of speech and language therapy services for children and young people. For this reason, local statistics which only report the *whole* population without considering all the different language and cultural communities should be treated with caution.
- Recognise that the national census is a snapshot undertaken at relatively long intervals. In the UK the national census is only undertaken every 10 years. Communities may change within that window. Changes to the local community, including differential birth rates, immigration, and movement both into and out of the area may therefore be missed by these reports. Consequently it is better to access local education department data and/or public health data, which are more likely to provide an accurate picture of the communities the profession aims to serve.
- Highlight reports and current themes emerging in the national press that apply to your local population(s) to flag up unmet needs to management and commissioners.

This may include reports on health inequalities, racism and other factors impacting on accessing services.

In addition to highlighting unmet needs, it is essential to highlight that at least double the amount of time is required to work with bilingual families compared to monolingual children (with whom you share a language). This is discussed earlier in the book. SLTs should emphasize that the professional organisations for SLTs, including RCSLT, ASHA, SPAA and IALP all recommend additional time when working with a family with whom you do not share a language.

Working outside your professional guidelines (for example by not providing sufficient contact time) may render you at risk of criticism, or even legal action. Should SLTs experience pressure to deviate from their professional clinical guidelines, it is recommended that the guidelines are presented to the supervising manager. If the supervising manager still insists on poor practice, then requesting a written exception and indemnity will likely prompt a re-evaluation of this stance. Although this may be considered provocative, the risk of being reported to the regulator (such as the Health and Care Professions Council) should not be underestimated.

## There are too many languages spoken in the local area so I will just work in the mainstream language (such as English)

This statement is often made by SLTs working in cities and large towns where hundreds of languages may be encountered. The feeling of being overwhelmed is understandable. However, a mainstream language approach will have negative outcomes for the child or young person and their family. Language attrition is highly likely to mean that the home language/mother tongue is lost, or significantly eroded, having long term sequalae for the bilingual child's mental health and wellbeing.

SLTs should be confident that they have the clinical skills and theoretical knowledge to provide a service in a language that they do not share with the family. This should be seen as a challenge, not a problem. Working through the processes described in this book constitute not only excellent service delivery, but opportunities for learning and development for the professional.

Regardless of your current level of clinical skill, working alongside an interpreter in home language is an opportunity to develop knowledge of that language. It is not essential that you are an expert on that particular language and culture. Continuing professional development (CPD) is a continuous process, and in choosing to take up this challenge you are meeting your professional standards.

## We don't have a specialist SLT in bilingualism

Although bilingualism is not a disorder, it is recommended that services encountering 10% or more referrals of bilingual families should develop a range of specialised roles. These might include:

- Specialist/Highly Specialist Speech and Language Therapist
- Consultant Speech and Language Therapist

Use the audit/data-based reports mentioned above to argue for funding for these roles.

Formal higher education should be considered by these post holders. Enquiry into speech, language, and communication disorders in a bilingual context, considering different communities and languages, is a fertile field for research.

SLTs aiming to develop expertise may wish to

- Take CPD short courses in bilingualism, for example a day's training led by an expert in the field
- Shadow a Specialist SLT in bilingualism
- Regularly attend a Clinical Excellence Network (CEN) or similar meeting of professionals with a special interest in bilingualism
- Attend or form a journal club to discuss and evaluate research papers and book chapters on bilingualism and how the findings might be applied to your own clinical practice
- Attend conferences, including not only those held by speech and language therapy professional bodies, but also those organised by other professional bodies such as linguistics and educational professionals
- Take short courses/post-graduate level units at university, such as a distance-learning course lasting 12 weeks
- Read books and published works to deepen your knowledge of themes mentioned in this book, such as codeswitching, bilingual phonology, or Developmental Language Disorder in languages other than English.

- Watch documentaries, listen to podcasts, and consume other multimedia by a specialist in bilingualism. Examples include:
    - Kletsheads Podcast (Unsworth, 2022)
    - Much Language Such Talk (Edinburgh University/Bilingualism Matters, 2022)

## The child needs X language for the education system so I have to deliver assessment and intervention in that language

As discussed in previous chapters, intervention in the mainstream language/language of education alone is not sufficient to help children overcome speech and language disorders. The evidence base is clear that, even for children with severe and complex needs (such as autistic spectrum conditions and learning difficulties) speech and language disorders are no bar to speaking home language/mother tongue. Further, assessment and intervention in the mainstream language only presents other risks which are not immediately obvious, such as threats to identity, cultural knowledge and good relationships with immediate family, the extended family and the community at large.

Understandably, parent(s)/carers are keen for their child to do well in the education system. This concern often overrides the need to maintain home language. Professionals may also believe that learning home language slows or prevents children and young people from acquiring an additional language (such as English). Such myths need to be dispelled.

To address the myth that children will only be successful in the education system if speech and language therapy is conducted in the language of that system the speech and language therapy team should not only discuss the evidence with the parent(s)/carer, but also educate the wider workforce around the child or young person.

This might include:

- Providing and/or writing information leaflets on typical bilingualism and on speech, language, and communication disorders in the context of bilingualism
- Training of the wider workforce on typical bilingualism and the advantages of bilingualism, as well as how best to support the use and maintenance of home language(s), even if the child or young person has a speech, language, or communication need
- Parent(s)/carer information sessions, where the evidence base can be presented in an accessible and jargon-free way. Highlighting to parent(s)/carers that children and young people need sufficient opportunities to use home language(s), and that they also

need to hear and converse in home language(s) on a daily basis. Choice of the language of education versus home language means that children will often lead by speaking the higher status mainstream language. Parent(s)/carers need consciously to set a home language usage policy for their home and may need support to think this through.

SLTs and education professionals would also do well to reflect on their own prejudices in relation to language learning and what they perceive as "the value" of a given language. While denying the rights of children from families to speak their home language these same people frequently express delight that their own children are being given the opportunity to learn another language at nursery or in the early years of the education system.

## If there is more than one home language spoken, which language(s) should assessment and therapy be delivered in?

For the assessment phase, *all* languages should be evaluated using a language case history and parental interview, as well as an appropriate battery of assessments.

The decision regarding in which language(s) to deliver intervention will flow from the assessment information and the desired outcome. The child or young person needs sufficient exposure to a particular language and opportunities to use that language. It is preferable if these opportunities cover a range of activities including play, conversation and daily household activities such as cooking.

For simultaneous acquisition of two or more languages in a household with each parent being the main speaker of a particular language, this may mean ensuring that each parent has sufficient time with the child to enable the above activities to take place. Brief interactions are unlikely to result in acquisition of that language, especially if the child has a speech or language disorder when more exposure may be required compared to a typically developing child.

As clinicians we have had many conversations with working fathers and working mothers who typically work full time and therefore have fewer opportunities for interaction with their children compared to the main carer. Some families may have grandparents as the main carer, while both parents work. It is a function of language acquisition that children speak the language they hear and use in everyday life. As much as a working parent might wish it, without sufficient interaction the child will at best become a receptive bilingual in that parent's language.

Parents therefore need to see their interaction patterns through the child's perspective and decide if they should:

- Divide child care so that parents both have sufficient opportunity to provide good models of their language
- Accept that they have insufficient opportunities with their child, and so prioritise formal language lessons in that language at a later stage when the child has acquired at least one of their home languages. The drawback with this approach is that they will not acquire this language when young and may therefore acquire it with an accent based on their home language phonology.

## I can't find a bilingual SLT or bilingual assistant/ co-worker to work with this particular family

Recruiting bilingual assistants and teaching assistants

Recruiting bilingual assistants by default, by adding the word "bilingual" to the job title, will attract a very different section of the workforce compared to using "Speech and Language Therapy Assistant" alone. Please see previous chapters on this topic.

When seeking personnel who speak a particular language, general recruitment strategies may not reach the community members you wish to employ. In this case, approaching local universities and colleges of higher education may yield overseas students attending their courses who speak the language(s) you need and will be willing to undertake part time employment. Such students will be taking a range of qualifications and it is worth approaching the establishment's employment services, posting job opportunities on notice boards and e-bulletins.

Local community centres may exist where members of the diaspora meet. Visiting these centres can also provide opportunities to recruit potential bilingual assistants.

All of these recruits should receive training on how to deliver the speech and language therapy intervention, as well being employed on a formal basis with accompanying mandatory training and check carried out prior to contact with children or young people.

As discussed earlier in this book it is unlikely that you will have a member of your team that speaks every language that you will encounter. SLTs should seek to use their phonological and linguistic knowledge to assess and devise intervention programmes in the home language(s) while working alongside an interpreter.

Prior to requesting an interpreter, bilingual assistant, teaching assistant, or other professional to deliver assessment and/or intervention, recall that it is imperative that the correct language is identified. Many families report the wrong language due to a range of complex factors. The only sure way is to check prior to the initial appointment using a three-way telephone call, or telehealth call. If the language reported does not match that spoken by the family, you will need to repeat this three-way interaction until the correct language/dialect is identified.

Implementing an intervention programme in school using the home language is challenging as the mainstream language is used almost exclusively by the adults and virtually mandated by the pragmatics of the setting. We have observed children reluctant to speak their home language even though they had little proficiency in the mainstream language/language of education. For this reason, a dedicated classroom assistant/teaching assistant who speaks the child or young person's home language is required to deliver the intervention programme and support them in the classroom should they need support.

Teaching assistants may also be subject to this embarrassment/reluctance to speak home language, even if paid to do so. Some communities are less familiar with adult-child interaction where the child takes the lead: they may expect adults to use directive language towards young children and do not view children as conversational partners. We have observed teaching assistants from some communities using home language to manage a child's behaviour, but not being confident enough to use home language for storytelling.

The teaching assistant may therefore need specific training on the use of home language in relation to facilitating children's initiations and interactions, if this is not part of the pragmatics of that community.

## I don't know anything about this particular language

Language acquisition theory, such as constructivism, is thought to be universal. The principles may be applied to any language. SLTs are unlikely to ever know about all languages spoken locally. However, on encountering a language for the first time, information and data on that language may be researched using key resources.

Speech sound inventories (phonological system) and language structure (syntax, grammar, phrase/word order and morphology) are available for a wide range of languages. These data may be found on:

- Professional bodies' web sites, such as RCSLT's Bilingualism Clinical Guidelines (RCSLT, 2019)
- Specialist publishers, such as Multilingual Matters
- Peer-reviewed journals and databases
- Teach yourself language guides and multimedia (Comrie, 2018)
- Language databases, such as Ethnologue

## I haven't got any assessments

As discussed earlier there are unlikely to be formal assessments in languages other than English. What few are available are growing, so it may be worth checking if one exists. Publishers are increasingly offering adaptations, or kits to help therapists to adapt existing assessments into other languages, taking into consideration linguistic, phonological and cultural differences. The major financial barrier to providing normative data is the collection, analysis and statistical processing of responses from typically developing children. Further, monolingual children will not acquire a particular language at the same rate, or in the same order or pattern, as children acquiring two or more languages.

Recall that informal assessments are equally as valid as formal assessments. Measuring the child against their own baseline using an approach such as the Dynamic Assessment Approach is best practice where standard assessments are unavailable.

Discuss with your local education colleagues that you will not be providing results in the form of standard scores, age equivalents, percentile ranks, or any other norm-referenced measure. In our experience, writing guidelines for gatekeepers of specialist provisions such as language resources/language units, additional support, and so forth are welcomed by education colleagues.

For example, a local language resource demanded that children perform at or below the 1st percentile for expressive language for access to the language unit provision. (A high staff to pupil ratio classroom within a mainstream school, with speech and language provision integrated into teaching for children with Developmental Language Disorder (DLD)). After explaining that using monolingual English norms to compare a bilingual child was not a valid approach, the agreed entry criteria was changed to the Specialist SLT in Bilingualism, stating "In my professional opinion [NAME] presents with Developmental Language Disorder and would benefit from intensive speech and language input."

## Conclusion

SLTs and other professionals can work effectively to provide appropriate and effective support to children experiencing speech, language, or communication disorders in a bilingual context. The professional, legal, and evidence-based clinical guidelines are clear that home language/mother tongue assessment and intervention are essential to good outcomes for the bilingual child or young person. Such services have been shown to be highly effective both in addressing the needs of the child and the acquisition or maintenance of home language skills. The benefits extend far wider than the family. Children and young people who maintain home language are able to fully engage with their family, extended family, and wider community and culture. Respect and dignity afforded to families will strengthen trust in professional services and in the profession.

We have found the intellectual and clinical challenges stimulating. Above all, our connections with families from a wide range of cultures and languages have enriched our lives and developed our sense of the diversity of human civilisation.

We have found working with bilingual families to be both fascinating and rewarding. We hope you do too. Bilingualism is an advantage!

## Resources

**Specialist publishers**
Multilingual Matters. www.multilingual-matters.com

**Language database**
Eberhard, D. M., Simons, G. F., & Fennig, C. D. (Eds.). (2022). *Ethnologue: Languages of the world* (25th ed.). SIL International. Online version www.ethnologue.com.

## References

Comrie, B. (Ed.). (2018). *The world's major languages* (3rd ed.). Routledge. ISBN 9780367580711.
Edinburgh University/Bilingualism Matters. (2022). *Much language such talk podcast*. https://www.mlstpodcast.com
Royal College of Speech and Language Therapists (RCSLT). (2019). *Clinical guidelines: Bilingualism*. www.rcslt.org.
Unsworth, S. (2022). *Kleitsheads [English edition]*. https://www.kletsheadspodcast.org

# RESOURCES

DOI: 10.4324/9781003125563-11

# QUIZZES

1. Speaking another language at home can slow down the acquisition of English, leading to a language delay.

    a. True

    b. False

2. A bilingual child can have typically developing home language and a language disorder in English.

    a. True

    b. False

3. A bilingual child can have a language disorder in their home language but not in English.

    a. True

    b. False

4. Codeswitching (using two languages in the same spoken sentence) is a sign of language confusion.

    a. True

    b. False

5. Stammering is more common in bilingual children.

    a. True

    b. False

6. Informal assessments such as describing culturally appropriate pictures is a better assessment for bilingual children than a published English language assessment.

    a. True

    b. False

7. In the UK, children have a legal right to speech and language therapy in their home language.

    a. True

    b. False

8. If a child has a severe language disorder, then parents should be advised to speak English only.

    a. True

    b. False

9. Parents should use one language only to avoid confusing children.

    a. True

    b. False

10. Which factor causes more Language Difficulties than the others?

    a. Bilingualism

    b. Lack of books in the home

    c. Deprivation/Poverty

    d. Prolonged dummy use after the age of 2 years

    e. Otitis media with effusion (Glue ear)

1. Speaking another language at home can slow down the acquisition of English, leading to a language delay.
   a. True
   b. **False**

   "Language Delay" is no longer used to describe children's Language Difficulties. It takes longer to learn two languages compared with one. However, the view that this causes a "delay," rather than seeing the bilingual language acquisition experience as *different* to monolingual language acquisition is inherently biased. The bilingual is not two monolingual speakers in one.

2. A bilingual child can have typically developing home language and a language disorder in English.
   a. True
   b. **False**

   A Language Difficulty (under the age of 5 years) or Developmental Language Disorder (DLD, age 5;0 or over, or before this age if likely to persist until after 5;0 years) will affect both/all languages spoken by the child or young person. If a child has acquired a first language successfully, then they have demonstrated that they can "break the code" (see Constructivist Language Acquisition theory). Any problems with additional language learning are therefore either a) a comparison to a monolingual English child, and therefore an unfair comparison; or a lack of sufficient opportunities to learn the additional language.

3. A bilingual child can have a language disorder in their home language but not in English.
   a. True
   b. **False**

   See above. Children and young people will have an underlying Developmental Language Disorder which will affect the acquisition of all their languages.

4. Codeswitching (using two languages in the same spoken sentence) is a sign of language confusion.
   a. True
   b. **False**

   Codeswitching is very frequent in most bilingual communities, although speakers may themselves view it negatively.

   Young children aged 3;6 and above rarely make errors in codeswitching. One language forms the frame or matrix, and content words (typically nouns and verbs) are inserted from any of the person's languages.

5. Stammering is more common in bilingual children.

    a. True

    b. **False**

    Dysfluency is the same in all populations. Bilingualism is not a demand on the child or young person. It is actually a capacity. The incidence of dysfluency is the same. However, some communities may not have a term or word for dysfluency and so may not recognises it as early. Late referrals, shame, or lack of awareness of dysfluency may contribute to this myth.

6. Informal assessments such as describing culturally appropriate pictures is a better assessment for bilingual children than a published English language assessment.

    a. **True**

    Since using standardised scores (percentile/centile ranks, age equivalents, standard deviations etc.) compares the child or young person to a monolingual child, they should not be applied to bilingual children. Similarly, cultural bias in the stimulus items (pictures, photos or toys and objects) may mean that the child fails some items as they are unfamiliar with them.

    Informal, culturally and linguistically adapted assessments are therefore more valid and should be used instead of standardised published formal assessments, unless they have been culturally and linguistically adapted.

    b. False

7. In the UK, children have a legal right to speech and language therapy in their home language.

    a. **True**

    The Equality Act (2010), and the Royal College of Speech and Language Therapists' Clinical Guidelines make it clear that clinicians must deliver assessment, advice and intervention in the home language.

    b. False

8. If a child has a severe language disorder, then parents should be advised to speak English only.

    a. True

    b. **False**

    Parent(s) and carers are likely to have their home language(s) as their best language. Children acquiring language need a complete language model. The best model for language acquisition is therefore the home language(s). Parents often wish to use the mainstream language (typically English) in order to support success in education. This myth must be robustly debunked.

9. Parents should use one language only to avoid confusing children.
   a. True
   b. **False**

   SLT should recommend speaking in the language which is that parent's strongest. This is the best language model for the child. However, recognise that codeswitching is a normal feature of most bilingual people's speech, and no attempt should be made to discourage it. Even families who try to adhere to one person one language approach are likely to codeswitch even though they themselves may not realise that they are doing so.

10. Which factor causes more Language Difficulties than the others?
   a. Bilingualism
   b. Lack of books in the home
   c. **Deprivation/Poverty**

   Deprivation affects nutrition, health, and educational attainment. Parent(s) and carers will often have grown up in deprivation themselves. The cycle of deprivation should be addressed at societal level. Social projects such as Head Start (US) and Sure Start (UK) are such initiatives.
   d. Prolonged dummy use after the age of 2 years
   e. Otitis media with effusion (Glue ear)

1. Speech Sound Disorder (SSD) is the diagnosis for children and young people with unclear speech.
   a. True
   b. False

2. If a child receives therapy for a phonological process (such as stopping) in one language, then this will generalise to both/all their languages.
   a. True
   b. False

3. If a child receives therapy for an articulation disorder in one language (such as a distortion), then this will generalise to both/all their languages.
   a. True
   b. False

4. A child may have Phonological Delay in their home language, and Consistent Phonological Disorder in their additional language (such as English).
   a. True
   b. False

5. A child may be able to use a phoneme in one language, but not another.
   a. True
   b. False

6. A child will have Inconsistent Phonological Disorder in both/all their languages.
   a. True
   b. False

7. Articulation disorder is defined as the inability to say a phoneme.
   a. True
   b. False

8. A bilingual child has a separate phonological system for each language they speak.
   a. True
   b. False

9. In languages other than English, phones such as /➜/ can start a word.
   a. True
   b. False

10. Bilingual children are more likely to experience Speech Sound Disorder than their monolingual peers.
    a. True
    b. False

1. Speech Sound Disorder (SSD) is the diagnosis for children and young people with unclear speech.
   a. True
   b. **False**

   SSD is a category, not a diagnostic label. It should be used as an overarching category, and prior to diagnosis as "suspected Speech Sound Disorder," with the precise diagnostic labels (such as "Articulation Disorder and Phonological Delay") used following assessment.

2. If a child receives therapy for a phonological process (such as stopping) in one language, then this will generalise to both/all their languages.
   a. True
   b. **False**

   Phonology is the mapping of meaning onto a speech code. This code is formed from contrasting units known as phonemes. If a process exists, it will affect one language differently to another since each language has a different contrastive system. Children may stop different fricatives, or not stop them at all in their other language.

3. If a child receives therapy for an articulation disorder in one language (such as a distortion), then this will generalise to both/all their languages.
   a. **True**

   Articulation of a single phone has no meaning. This is a physical production. If the phone is used in both/all languages, then accuracy in forming the physical articulation within the vocal tract will be available to both/all languages.
   b. False

4. A child may have Phonological Delay in their home language, and Consistent Phonological Disorder in their additional language (such as English).
   a. True
   b. **False**

   The underlying phonological disorder (Phonological Delay, Consistent Phonological Disorder; Inconsistent Phonological Disorder) will be present in both/all languages. However, the surface patterns may be different in each language.

5. You may hear a child say a phoneme in one language, but not another.
   a. True
   b. **False**

Children may have *word level* phonological processes that differ between languages, and so you may hear a child realise a phoneme (as a phone) in one language and not another.

6. A child will have Inconsistent Phonological Disorder in both/all their languages.
   a. **True**

      Inconsistent Phonological Disorder is identified by a very high variability in the production of *words* on different occasions (not phones or phonemes). There is essentially no mapping onto word templates for any language.
   b. False

7. Articulation disorder is defined as the inability to say a phoneme.
   a. True
   b. **False**

      Phonemes are psycholinguistic units of contrast, concerned with the production of words. Articulation disorder is when the realisation of phones leads to distortion, or the incorrect phone being realised as a single sound, or in Consonant + Vowel (CV), Vowel + Consonant (VC) or CVC combinations, *provided* that these CV, VC and CVC combinations are not real words in either language (as that would invoke phonology).

8. A bilingual child has a separate phonological system for each language they speak.
   a. **True**

      There is one contrastive system for each language, but only one vocal tract.
   b. False

9. In languages other than English, phones such as /ŋ/can start a word.
   a. **True**

      The phonotactics of a language (which sounds may appear in which word and syllable position) are different across languages. Some languages such as English do not allow a voiced velar nasal to start a word or syllable. Other languages such as Urdu, a Pakistani-heritage language, do, in words such as "watch"/ŋkʰʌɾi /
   b. False

10. Bilingual children are more likely to experience Speech Sound Disorder than their monolingual peers.
    a. True
    b. **False**

       There is no reason why children who speak two or more languages should experience Speech Sound Disorder more frequently than monolingual children. However, late identification and referral may lead to a greater impact of SSD on bilingual children.

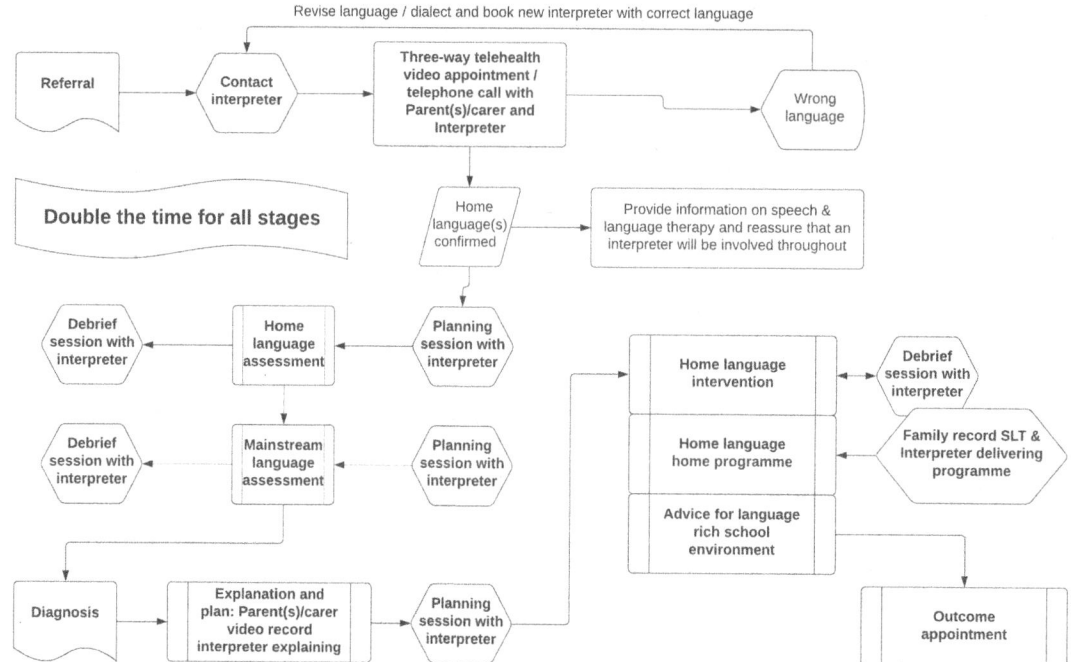

**Figure 11.1** Care Pathway when working with bilingual families

# CASE STUDIES

The following are brief case studies taken from clinical practice. The children and young people's names have been changed and some details altered to protect anonymity. By definition such examples are simplistic and lacking in detail but are often helpful to contextualise learning in the context of a real service user and family. The case studies are presented here for use by students, speech and language therapy teams and other professionals to reflect on how the concepts and principles set out in this book should be applied in real life clinical settings.

Mehboob comes from a home where both Mirpuri and English are spoken. Mirpuri has no written form. Mehreen, Mehboob's mother speaks Mirpuri and only speaks a few phrases in English. Mehreen is a full-time mother and enjoys meeting with other Mirpuri speaking mothers and the extended family. Zeeshan, Mehboob's father, speaks both Mirpuri and English. Zeeshan uses English daily as he works in an English-speaking environment. Zeeshan mainly speaks English to the family.

Mehboob has an older brother, Iqbal (aged 7;2) who speaks Mirpuri and English fluently. The family live in an area of socio-economic deprivation in the North West of England.

Mehboob has no expressive language and uses only crying, open vowels verbally. Mehboob uses pointing and eye pointing to communicate his needs. Mehboob becomes very frustrated and his mother reports that there are long periods when Mehboob cries and kicks the door.

Mehboob cooperated well with toy and picture book assessments. His receptive vocabulary and verbal comprehension in Mirpuri are age appropriate. Mehboob only recognises a few words (nouns) in English. Mehboob is stimulable for a range of single sounds including nasals [m], [n]; plosives [p], [b], [t] and long vowels. Mehboob can select pictures from a choice of three on request in Mirpuri, such as:

| Mirpuri utterance | dzanani | axbar | par-ni pi |
|---|---|---|---|
| Morpheme-by-morpheme direct translation | Lady | newspaper | read-ing + female is + female |
| Nearest English equivalent | Show me "(the) lady (she) is reading (a) newspaper" | | |

Mehboob has been referred to the Community Paediatrician, Audiology, and a Children's Centre. His listening and attention skills are well developed. Mehboob has mild otitis media with effusion, but this is not sufficient to explain his speech and Language Difficulties. He is otherwise well, and his gross and fine motor development are age appropriate. Mehboob has now been referred to a geneticist.

1. What is Mehboob's speech and language diagnosis?
2. Is action indicated?
3. What intervention is proposed?
4. What service delivery model should be followed?
5. How will intervention be evaluated?

1.  Mehboob has significant speech and Language Difficulties which interfere with his ability to express his basic needs and to interact with his family and children of his age.

    The fact that Mehboob has an older brother who is a fluent bilingual speaker rules out environmental causes such as severe deprivation.

    Mehboob's problems affect his output, as his listening vocabulary and receptive skills are typical for a child of his age.

    The comorbidity of a severe Speech Sound Disorder (SSD) is unsurprising as many children with language disorder also experience SSD (Broomfield & Dodd, 2004).

    Mehboob's frustration is directly attributable to his communication disorder.

    Mehboob's willingness to cooperate with unfamiliar adults for assessment of these skills suggests good interaction and social skills.

    Mehboob presents with Language Difficulty or Speech, Language, and Communication Needs (SLCN). Mehboob is likely to be diagnosed with Developmental Language Disorder (DLD) if he does not make significant progress in the next year or so.

2.  A child of this age should easily be able to express his needs and more. Mehboob cannot use any word combinations in any of his languages. Nor can Mehboob produce a codeswitched simple utterance such as an AGENT + ACTION or AGENT + PATIENT + ACTION combination (McKean et al., 2013).

    Mehboob requires urgent, intensive intervention to develop his expressive language skills and his speech skills.

3.  Mehboob should be offered intensive speech and language therapy with daily input. Mehboob is past the age of a "late talker" (Reilly et al., 2018) and unlikely to resolve without immediate action.

    Mehboob should receive intervention in his home language of Mirpuri. Failure to develop his home language skills will mean that he is isolated from his mother. The likely impact of an English-only approach would be to isolate Mehboob from his immediate family and community, likely causing psychological and emotional harm.

4.  Resources such as a language unit or specialist provision should be considered. A classroom assistant who speaks Mirpuri and English should be employed to support Mehboob in the classroom situation and deliver his speech and language therapy programme. While this is arranged, 2–3 times weekly input in clinic with the assistance of an interpreter would be appropriate.

5.  The best outcome for Mehboob would be for him to achieve age-appropriate expressive language and speech sound skills in his home language. This would mean that he will be able to acquire English from his educational exposure.

*Outcome*

Mehboob was referred to the local language unit where he was supported by a classroom assistant in Mirpuri and a Specialist SLT who designed expressive language and speech sound therapy aims in Mirpuri using the available data on the language (Pert, 2007; Stow, 2006; Stow & Pert, 2006). A member of the team suggested AAC or signing as a way of helping Mehboob communicate. However, he made sufficient progress in the first episode of care to indicate that a verbal approach would be possible. Mehboob was provided with regular small group and individual speech and language therapy sessions in home language only, while attending an English-medium education setting.

Mehboob was found to have a genetic condition not previously linked to Language Disorder. Subsequent investigations found further cases, and this has now been documented in the literature.

Mehboob was discharged just over two years after referral with fully intelligible and well-formed, age-appropriate Mirpuri language skills. Mehboob acquired English language skills without any specific targets in his speech and language therapy through usual additional language learning. The teaching staff commented that Mehboob quickly acquired the English language skills after practicing a similar concept or construction in his home language. Mehboob was discharged and did not require any further treatment for his speech and language skills through to adulthood.

Mehboob's parents commented that his ability to use and understand his home language, as well as English, meant that he had achieved the same skills as his older brother. Mehboob was able to participate in family gatherings and speak to relatives with confidence in both home language and English.

Maria has been referred by her mother due to concerns about her talking. Maria's mother is Brazilian and so Maria comes from a home where both Portuguese and English are spoken. Maria's father is English, and he speaks both languages but prefers English. Maria's older brother Lucas (aged 10;5) speaks both languages fluently. There is no history of speech and Language Difficulties in the family. The parents had been trying to use a one-person one-language approach and are pleased that this appears to be working. They are now however so worried about Maria's language skills that they are considering just using English at home as they feel bilingual input is confusing Maria.

Maria has well-developed symbolic play skills and enjoys a range of activities with other children her age. Maria's listening and attention are age appropriate. There are no developmental concerns.

Maria has basic sentences in Portuguese but has difficulty understanding and using adjectives, verb tenses and other language features. Maria rarely codeswitches.

Maria's English is limited despite two years in educational settings. Maria can understand a range of nouns and a limited number of high frequency verbs.

Maria's speech sound development is very limited in Portuguese. Maria is only able to use nasals and plosives. There is no vowel distortion. In English, Maria is able to use a range of sounds including nasals, plosives and fricatives.

Maria has no hearing impairment, and her development is not a cause for concern.

1. What is Maria's speech and language diagnosis?
2. Is action indicated?
3. What advice would you give to Maria's parents about their language choices?
4. What intervention(s) are proposed?
5. What service model will be followed?

1. Maria has significant Language Difficulties in both her home languages, Portuguese and English, despite sufficient exposure and opportunities for play-based learning. Since Maria's brother had no difficulties acquiring both languages, it is unlikely that the parents' input is the cause of these difficulties. Maria is likely to reach the age of 5 before she can resolve these difficulties, and therefore Developmental Language Disorder (DLD) should be diagnosed now. Maria also has Speech Sound Disorder (SSD) and this is not unusual as many children with DLD also have other domains of speech, language, and communication affected.

2. Maria needs urgent speech and language therapy. Maria's difficulties are unlikely to resolve without intervention. It is worth noting that Maria's mother considered the bilingualism to be the cause of Maria's problems, despite the fact that her son had no such issues. This was probably due to the negative attitude of Maria's teacher towards her bilingualism. Intervention should be in the home language, as, although both parents have access to English, Maria's family have significant family and emotional ties with Brazil. Maria would be expected to live with relatives for extended holidays and it is important for Maria's identity and awareness of her own culture that she be able to speak Portuguese.

3. Maria's parents had adopted a one-person one-language approach. This approach can be useful if one parent is the sole source of a language. However, since both parents speak both Portuguese and English, it is likely that they codeswitch whether they are aware of this or not. Even if they do not codeswitch, the stated reason for segregating the languages, to avoid confusion, is not supported by the literature. Maria's parents were therefore encouraged to use Portuguese as the main home language (since this was the sole source of input for Maria) and English outside the home. The exceptions were when an English-language topic was being discussed, such as English homework, or when English-speaking visitors came to the home.

4. Maria requires intervention for both her language skills and her speech. Intervention was devised in home language using available normative data on Brazilian Portuguese (McLeod, 2007; Pires et al., 2011; Valian & Eisenberg, 1996). Maria's mother was keen to engage in Portuguese language therapy activities.

   Since Maria's teacher had commented that Maria's bilingualism and different culture may have caused or contributed to her speech and language disorder, a training session was arranged for teachers at the school on bilingualism and speech, language, and communication needs. This approach meant that the individual teacher was not highlighted and that other bilingual children attending the school would also avoid having any SLCN attributed to their bilingualism.

5. In the local area, Brazilian Portuguese was not spoken by many families. For this reason, individual therapy at clinic with the assistance of an interpreter was selected, rather than a small group. A referral to the Language Unit for intensive intervention was made, but the resource was full at this time and Maria's parents preferred her to stay with her current classmates.

*Outcome*

Maria needed several episodes of care to achieve conversational and narrative skills in Portuguese. Maria's English progressed in terms of syntax and grammar, but she still made mistakes and needed more exposure and opportunities to try out new structures than her bilingual peers. In common with many children and young people with DLD, Maria's problems continued throughout her educational career, but at a sub-clinical level.

Maria's parents were pleased with her progress and came to terms with the fact that Maria would have experienced DLD and Speech Sound Disorder if she had been raised in a monolingual or bilingual environment.

Peter has been referred by his father with concerns about his speech sounds. Peter's mother is an English-Cantonese speaker of Chinese heritage, and his father is an English speaker of English heritage. Peter's mother uses Cantonese for stories and some social occasions but mainly uses English with Peter. Peter's father only speaks English to Peter. Peter's father is concerned that Peter's "r" sound is odd and that this has been caused by his mother's use of Cantonese. He has therefore asked his wife to stop using Cantonese at home.

Peter is healthy, and there are no concerns about his hearing or development. Peter is doing well at school and considered a bright pupil. Peter's listening and attention is age appropriate.

Peter's English language skills, vocabulary, and naming are in the moderately high range. Peter's *Diagnostic Evaluation of Articulation and Phonology* (DEAP) (Dodd et al., 2002) shows no speech errors except /ɹ/➜[w]. Peter has age-appropriate scores on the *Preschool and Primary Inventory of Phonological Awareness* (PIPA) (Dodd et al., 2000) and his literacy skills are developing faster than his peers.

1.  What is Peter's speech and language diagnosis?
2.  Is action indicated?
3.  What advice would you give to Peter's parents?
4.  What intervention is proposed?
5.  How would you measure the success of the intervention (outcome?)

1. Peter is essentially a monolingual English speaker. Peter had some very minimal familiarity with Cantonese, but no functional understanding or use of the language. Monolingual English phonetic acquisition norms show that the voiced alveolar approximant is not acquired by 90% of children until the age of 6 to 6 and a half years (Dodd et al., 2003). At word level, the phonological process of gliding persists until the age of 5;11 (see Appendix). Since Peter is only 5;6 years, neither the acquisition of the phone, nor the suppression of the simplification pattern can be assumed. Peter therefore has age-appropriate speech.

2. No. Treatment is not indicated since there are no errors which are not frequently observed in the majority of the population at this age. There is no reason to believe that Peter will not acquire /ɹ/ at sound level and supress gliding at word level at the appropriate age, as shown by the normative data.

3. Peter's parents were shown the normative data and reassured that Peter's speech was entirely normal for his age. They were invited to re-refer Peter after the age of 6;6 if he were still unable to use the target sound.

4. None.

5. Peter's father's concern was motivated by unconscious internalised racism. He blamed an apparent speech disorder on the presence of a minimal amount of a language other than English. This perception that bilingual is harmful is still sadly commonly encountered. Even if Peter had presented with a Speech Sound Disorder, the aetiology (underlying cause) would not have been exposure to another language.

Aleena comes from a home where Mirpuri and Punjabi, Pakistani-heritage languages, are spoken. Aleena's mother speaks Mirpuri, and her father speaks Punjabi. Aleena has been referred by the Health Visitor following concerns that Aleena is only using single words. Aleena lives in a town in North West England, which is an area of socio-economic deprivation. Aleena's father is a taxi driver, and Aleena's mother is a housewife. Aleena has a younger brother aged 2;0 and two older sisters, aged 4;1 and 6;2. Both older sisters were referred to speech and language therapy but were discharged for non-attendance. Aleena still uses a dummy (pacifier) and has an extensive open-bite malocclusion (See Verrastro et al., 2006). Aleena eats normally but still likes two bottles of milk fed to her before bedtime. The family are not concerned and say that she is too young to speak properly yet and that her sisters were just the same. They say they would not have referred Aleena and don't want to have to come to clinic as they are very busy with all the children.

Aleena has been referred to Audiology and has no hearing difficulties. Aleena's development is within normal limits. Assessment in Mirpuri shows that Aleena can understand spoken instructions in the same way as her peers. Aleena's naming is limited to everyday nouns and basic verbs such as "eating," "drinking," "washing," and "walking." Aleena does not combine word together. Aleena's phonology is limited to nasals and plosives, although Aleena is stimulable for fricatives at sound level (stimulable).

1. What is Aleena's speech and language diagnosis?
2. Is action indicated?
3. What intervention is proposed?
4. What advice would you give to Aleena's parents?
5. How will the intervention be evaluated?

1.  Aleena has a Language Difficulty or SLCN. There is a family history of Language Difficulty, with a complex range of contributing factors, including social deprivation, possible genetic predisposition to Language Difficulties (although it is impossible to unravel environmental and genetic factors here), and lack of concern by parents. This lack of concern may be troubling to professionals. However, parents may compare their child to siblings (or neighbour's or extended family peers) rather than use objective measures. Beliefs about language development, causes of Language Difficulties and possible interventions may differ from white English-speaking communities (Marshall et al., 2017).

    The lack of contrast in Aleena's phonological system cannot be attributed solely to her open bite malocclusion. Aleena has a Phonological Delay affecting her home language, which will be evident in her English when she begins education.

    Aleena is a monolingual speaker in a language other than English and is expected to become bilingual in the future, via attendance at an educational setting.

2.  Yes. Intervention is required, delivered in Aleena's home language. Without home language(s), Aleena will not be able to communicate with her parents and extended family.

3.  Language and speech sound intervention is required in home language(s).

4.  It may be tempting to recommend a Parent-Child Interaction Therapy approach for a child with this kind of Language Difficulty. However, there are cultural barriers to this approach. Many families find engaging in this style of input problematic and prefer more direct approaches (see Awde, 2009). A language intervention approach where languages other than English are possible such as the *Building Early Sentence Therapy* (BEST) may be more suitable (McKean et al., 2013).

5.  The clinician might wish to use a Dynamic Assessment approach, comparing both the range of language structures and the Mean Length of Utterance after an episode of care with Aleena's initial language presentation.

Badal comes from a family where Sylheti Bengali and English are spoken. Badal's mother speaks Sylheti, and his father speaks Sylheti and English. Badal has been receiving speech and language therapy episodes of care with consolidation breaks since he was referred aged 3;6 and diagnosed with Developmental Language Disorder (DLD). Badal has an Educational Health and Care Plan (EHCP) (Department for Education, 2022) which identified funding for 4 hours a day one-to-one classroom support in Sylheti. Badal has progressed well in therapy, which was delivered in Sylheti by a bilingual speech and language therapy assistant and a bilingual classroom assistant.

Badal is able to use his expressive language skills to access his lessons in class and is doing very well academically, especially in maths. Badal is also speaking Sylheti well at home and uses it to converse with the extended family. Badal is however having difficulty making and maintaining friends at school. His father is concerned that Badal is reporting that he is lonely at school and that other children ignore him.

Badal is reported by his classroom assistant and teacher to relate well to supportive adults but that with other children he does not initiate conversation. Badal can use question words in assessment conditions.

1. What is Badal's communication profile?
2. Is action indicated?
3. What intervention is proposed?
4. What language(s) should the intervention be delivered in?

1. Badal has an established diagnosis (DLD) and care package in place. This support is effective, and he is developing both his home language (Sylheti) and mainstream language (English) skills. However, this is always with supportive adults. Some, but not all children with DLD have difficulties with peer relationships. Badal needs to use his developing language skills to initiate and maintain friendships.

2. Yes. Intervention should be holistic and consider the functions of language, as well as capability. This includes peer relationships.

3. Focusing on play and encouraging social skills are likely to be protective against mental health problems in the future (Toseeb et al., 2020). A buddying scheme might be considered. Such schemes have been shown to increase interactions for both typically developing children and children with autism/autistic children (Morrier & Ziegler, 2018).

4. Badal's peers in the school setting will likely use the mainstream language. However, outside of school, Badal may be more likely to socialise with siblings, neighbours and those from his language community. The clinician will need to consider that pragmatics may differ, as well as the games and activities that are favoured in each community.

Zeeshan comes from a home where Mirpuri, a Pakistani-heritage language, and English are spoken. Zeeshan was referred by his mother as he "sounds unclear." Zeeshan's parents both speak Mirpuri and English, but speak mainly Mirpuri to Zeeshan at home. They are concerned that he is mixing up sentences in both languages and that this confusion will slow down his language development.

On assessment Zeeshan does use English and Mirpuri words together. You observe him saying the following (transliterated by the interpreter):

| Child's utterance 1 | *girl* | *chair* | uper | beh-ti vi |
|---|---|---|---|---|
| Morpheme-by-morpheme translation | girl | chair | on | sit-ing + female is + female |
| Nearest English translation | (the) girl is sitting on (a) chair ||||
| Target Mirpuri utterance | *kuri kursi* uper beh-ti vi <br> girl chair on sit-ing + female is + female ||||

| Child's utterance 2 | the *dzanani* | is cooking | *chavel* |
|---|---|---|---|
| Morpheme-by-morpheme translation | the *woman/lady* | is cooking | *rice* |
| Nearest English translation | The *lady/woman* is cooking *rice* |||
| Target Mirpuri utterance | dzanani chavel peka-ni pi <br> lady/woman rice cook-ing + female is + female |||

| Child's utterance 3 | meh | *banana* | passanda |
|---|---|---|---|
| Morpheme-by-morpheme translation | I | banana | like |
| Nearest English translation | I like (the) banana |||
| Target Mirpuri utterance | meh *kela* passanda <br> I *banana* like |||

| Child's utterance 4 | *boy* | *jump* mar-na pi-ja |
|---|---|---|
| Morpheme-by-morpheme translation | boy | *jump* do-ing + male + contact is + male |
| Nearest English translation | (the) boy (he) is *jumping* ||
| Target Mirpuri utterance | *mura charl* mar-na pi-ja <br> boy jump do-ing + male +contact is + male ||

| Child's utterance 5 | eh mura | *flower* | *smell* kar-na pi-ja |
|---|---|---|---|
| Morpheme-by-morpheme translation | this boy | *flower* | *smell* do-ing + male is + male |
| Nearest English translation | this boy (he) is smelling (a) flower | | |
| Target Mirpuri utterance | eh mura *phul sung*-ena pi-ja<br>this boy flower smell-ing + male is + male | | |

Considering that Mirpuri is a language where the word/phrase order is AGENT + OBJECT + ACTION (or *Subject + Object = Verb* SOV in surface form terminology), are Zeeshan's utterances unusual?

1. What is Zeeshan's speech and language diagnosis?
2. What advice would you give Zeeshan's parents?
3. Is action required?

1.  Zeeshan is codeswitching within an utterance. This is known as intrasentential codes-witching. This type of codeswitching, where one language sets the syntactic frame and the content words (typically nouns and verbs) are inserted from any of the languages known to the speaker, is typical of bilingual speakers from the British Pakistani-heritage community.

    Adult speakers are likely to view codeswitching as "sloppy" or "imperfect." However, Zeeshan is following the AGENT + PATIENT + ACTION phrase order for his Mirpuri utterances in examples i), iii), iv), and v). Zeeshan is following the English phrase order AGENT + ACTION + PATIENT in example ii).

    Zeeshan therefore has adult-style codeswitching and no difficulties with either Mirpuri or English (See Myers-Scotton, 2002; Pert & Letts, 2006).

    Zeeshan does not require a diagnosis.

2.  To encourage Zeeshan to speak both his home language, Mirpuri, and his mainstream language, English in the same way as he has always done.

3.  No. Zeeshan can be discharged as treatment is not indicated.

Daniyal comes from a home where Punjabi is spoken. Daniyal was referred by his parents after concerns that he was not talking clearly. Daniyal's mother has only lived in the UK for five years after marrying Daniyal's father. As Daniyal's mother looks after the family, she spends most of her time at home and with relatives and has not picked up as much English as she would like to.

As Daniyal is starting school his mother is trying to use as much English as possible to help him to be confident. She has switched from using only Punjabi, to using only English in the last six months to achieve this aim.

Daniyal is very quiet at the assessment session. When he does attempt to speak, he looks down and talks very quietly. He cooperates with a receptive language assessment but doesn't speak when asked to name or cooperate with an expressive language task. His receptive language is above average for his age in Punjabi.

He speaks to the bilingual assistant to ask to go to the toilet in Punjabi. You decide to leave Daniyal to play with the assistant while you and his mother observe through a one-way mirror. During play with Lego Daniyal repeats the first word of each spoken sentence between one and three times but does not appear to be aware of this.

1. What is Daniyal's speech and language diagnosis likely to be?
2. What advice can you give to his parents?
3. What actions would you recommend?

1. Daniyal is hearing a limited language model from his main carer, his mother. English is not her strongest and most complete language, and her mother tongue would be a better model for Daniyal.

   It is possible that Daniyal has limited expressive language.

   it is also possible that Daniyal has dysfluent speech (stammering/stuttering). His mother may not know about stammering/stuttering or have no word for the condition.

2. Daniyal's mother speaks Punjabi fluently. This language is the best model for Daniyal. Since English is also used, a codeswitched version would also be a naturalistic language model. The family should be advised to use Punjabi as their main home language as this will enhance Daniyal's language acquisition. It is also likely that unless Punjabi is used at home, Daniyal will experience language attrition and be unable to speak Punjabi with his mother in the future. This may interfere with their relationship, as Daniyal's mother has limited English language skills.

3. Further assessment of expressive language and fluency is indicated.

Aadil has been referred by his parents because he sounds unclear in his home language (Mirpuri). The family speak Mirpuri and English and Aadil has three older brothers, none of whom had any speech or Language Difficulties.

You carry out a *Diagnostic Evaluation of Articulation and Phonology* (DEAP) (Dodd et al., 2002) in English. Aadil's speech sounds are all in place in his single-word production, with the exception of /θ/ ➔ [f] and /ð/ ➔ [v]. Aadil is also not stimulable for these phones when asked to produce them in isolation. Aadil omits the first segment /s/ from word initial tri-clusters, but not di-clusters. He is stimulable for [s].

Aadil's language skills are all above average.

When feeding back the assessment results to Aadil's parents they insist that his /k/ is produced as [t] in Mirpuri. They give the examples of "kuri" (girl) and "kela" (banana). On your DEAP assessment, Aadil produced all /k/ phonemes on target in English. Furthermore, Aadil can readily imitate [t] and [k] as single phones in isolation.

1.  What is Aadil's likely diagnosis?
2.  What actions would you take?

1. The dental fricatives are not acquired in English until the age of 7 or above.

   The reduction of tri-clusters by omitting a segment is a simplification pattern (phonological process) found in the speech of younger children. This phonological process is usually supressed by 90% of children by the age of 4;11 years (Dodd et al., 2003). Aadil therefore has Phonological Delay in English.

   Aadil has phonological errors in his Mirpuri contrastive system that do not occur in English, and vice versa. The fact that Aadil is stimulable for both the voiceless alveolar plosive and the voiceless velar plosive show that this is not an articulation disorder.

   Aadil's preliminary diagnosis of Speech Sound Disorder (SSD) can now be narrowed down to Phonological Delay. This is evident in both of his languages, albeit with different surface patterns in each one; velar fronting in Mirpuri, and tri-cluster reduction in English.

   The phonological simplification process of fronting should be eliminated in Mirpuri-English children after the age of 4;11 (Stow & Pert, 2020).

2. A full phonological assessment in Mirpuri will confirm the above diagnosis.

   Aadil's errors in Mirpuri need to be addressed at word level and above in both his languages, using a meaning-based (phonological) approach.

# CALCULATING THE AGE OF DIVERSE CHILDREN AND YOUNG PEOPLE FOR THE APPLICATION OF NORMATIVE DATA: WHEN IS IT APPROPRIATE?

## Developing skills

Since children are developing their speech and language skills towards a complete adult system, older children tend to have more developed skill levels than do younger children. However, there are individual differences, and just like any other human skill or attribute, speech and language development are distributed across the normative range. This range is represented using a normal distribution curve (or "bell curve") for a particular population.

For most speech and language disorders, it is not a binary "disorder present" versus "disorder not present" decision. Children and young people may have some areas of relative strength and some areas of relative need. For this reason, different *domains* may be considered separately, as well as the overall speech and language skills.

Domains for language include receptive language skills (verbal comprehension), expressive language skills (constructing grammatically and morphologically well-formed and acceptable utterances), listening vocabulary (receptive word knowledge), and naming. Domains for speech include acquisition of phones (articulation skills), inventory of phonemes acquired and used appropriately in words, presence and elimination of phonological processes, and phonological awareness skills. These are not exhaustive lists.

Additionally, a bilingual child's skills in one language are unlikely to be matched by their skills in their other language(s), and normative data are unlikely to be available for the very wide range and variation of language exposure between individuals in a bilingual population.

## Converting the child's performance on this assessment to a format in which we can compare their performance to other children of their age and cultural and linguistic background

"Raw scores," the actual number of correct responses on a particular standardised test or assessment, tell us nothing about how well a particular child has achieved *compared to other children of their age.* To make a meaningful comparison, we need to convert the raw score to a standard score and then map that score onto the normal distribution curve.

## Cut-off below which the child's performance is considered impaired or disordered

Different domains may be "mapped" onto the normal distribution curve. There is no overall agreement as to where disorder emerges. Some clinicians consider anything below one standard deviation away from the mean to be clinically significant (–1.0 or below, or < 16th percentile), whilst other clinicians consider –1.5 standard deviations below the mean to be the limit.

## Strengths and problems of this approach

The strength of this approach is that the clinician can be confident that the child is or is not performing in the same way as their peers.

The problem with these calculations is that most assessments are standardised on white monolingual English-speaking populations. Applying these standardised scores to a child who does not have English as their home language is unfair and an example of institutionalised racism. This is why **children speaking languages other than English (LOTE) should *never* be compared to English monolingual children using standard deviations, standard scores, percentiles/percentile ranks, centile, age equivalents, or other similar data,** unless the standardisation data were collected from a bilingual population that has a similar life experience and language exposure to the child or young person being assessed.

Cultural differences will also invalidate such assessments, as children may be unfamiliar with the assessment materials or assessment method, and so fail to provide the expected response even though they may have acquired the skill to do so if they were assessed in a more culturally appropriate manner.

For these reasons, when working with diverse populations the following key approaches are employed instead of using assessments standardised on monolingual (mainly white) populations:

- **Using an assessment developed for the specific population**
  Examples include the Bilingual Speech Sound Screen (BiSSS; Stow & Pert, 2019), which has normative data collected from Pakistani-heritage children who are sequential bilinguals (Pakistani-heritage languages and English). Note that BiSSS would not be

appropriate for either monolingual Mirpuri/Punjabi/Urdu speakers living in Pakistan, or monolingual English speakers living in the UK.

- **Using a descriptive or Dynamic Assessment Approach**
  These approaches describe the child or young person's strengths and needs, rather than focusing on age of acquisition.

- **Using a formal assessment descriptively**
  Although this avoids using the normative data collected on another population, it still does not address the cultural bias of the pictures/objects and the problems encountered when translating questions and tasks from one language to another.

If you are employing an assessment which includes normative data from the same population as the child or young person, then you are likely to need the child's age on assessment.

## Calculating completed years, months (and days)

To calculate a child's age, we aim to calculate the number of years and completed months. This is the standard way in which assessment tables are constructed.

Please note that the UK date format is referred to throughout these examples.

1. List the date of assessment in reverse UK order: YYYY/MM/DD.
2. List the child or young person's date of birth in reverse UK order below the date of assessment.
3. Subtract the day of birth from the day of assessment.
   a. If there are insufficient days, then borrow 31 days and reduce the month by 1.
4. Subtract the month of birth from the month of assessment.
   a. If there are insufficient months, then borrow 12 months and reduce the year by 1.
5. Subtract the year of birth from the year of assessment.
6. Format the result as YY;MM.DD

## Examples

Consider a child born on 3 August 2018 and assessed on 4 September 2022.

| Date of assessment: | 2022/09/04 |
| --- | --- |
| Date of birth: | 2018/08/03 |
| Age in years and completed months: | 4;1.1 |

*which is 4 years, 1 month, and 1 day old.* Cite this age in reports as **4;1 years.**

Consider a child born on 28 May 2019 and assessed on 17 March 2022.

| Date of assessment: | 2022/03/17 |
|---|---|
| Date of birth: | 2019/05/28 |
| Age in years and completed months: | **2;9**.20 |

Cite this age in reports as **2;9 years.**

## DAYS

28 from 17 won't go, so we borrow one month, or 31 days, from "'03," which becomes "02." (31 + 17) – 28 = 20 days

## MONTHS

05 from 02 won't go (recall that we borrowed one month in the step above), so we borrow one year, or 12 months, from "2022," which becomes "2021." (02 + 12) – 05 = 9 months

## YEARS

2021 – 2019 = 2 years (recall that we borrowed one year in the step above).

**Notes**

- Most assessments do not pay attention to the number of completed days, and so children and young people's ages are mainly reported in years;months (YY;MM).

- Providing age in YY;MM format is only applicable to children and young people. This format should not be used for adults (unless stated in the assessment manual).

- If you do not like this method, or if you do these calculations frequently, you may wish to automate the calculation using a spreadsheet. The formula for Microsoft® Excel is:
  - **Years** difference between two dates: DATEDIF (Cell01, Cell02, "Y")
  - **Months** difference between two dates: DATEDIF (Cell01, Cell02, "YM")
  - **Or use the spreadsheet provided.**

| D.O.B. (dd/mm/yyyy): | | | |
|---|---|---|---|
| Date of assessment (dd/mm/yyyy): | | | |
| Age on assessment: | Enter Date of Birth; | or | months |
| | | | |

## Reference

Stow, C. and Pert, S. (2020). *Bilingual Speech Sound Screen (BiSSS): Revised and expanded edition.* The University of Manchester, UK. https://estore.manchester.ac.uk/product-catalogue/faculty-of-biology-medicine-and-health/school-of-health-sciences/bilingual-speech-sound-screen-bisss/bilingual-speech-sound-screen-bisss

## Speech Sound Disorder and the bilingual child

*Notes for the Speech and Language Therapist/Pathologist:*

☑ Please ask an interpreter to provide the following information in the family's home language(s).

☑ Consider that some technical terms including "sound," "word," "vocal tract," etc., may not have translation equivalents and will need examples to explain these clearly. Discuss these in the planning session before you discuss the diagnosis with the family.

☑ With permission from the interpreter, video and/or audio record the interpreter delivering this information in home language(s) and upload the recording so that it is available online (generic information leaflets are not confidential information).

☑ Link the web address to a QR code and add it here with the language(s) available for quick access by the parent(s)/carer and family via a camera on a smartphone or tablet.

## What is speech?

Speech is made up of different sounds. Most sounds are made using parts of the mouth such as the lips, teeth, tongue and other parts of the vocal tract. The voice box (larynx) makes a buzzing noise for loud sounds. We use speech to speak out loud so that others can hear us, listen and understand what we are saying. The sound waves move through the air from the speaker's mouth to the listener's ears.

**Speech** means the sounds we make. **Language** is the meaning of the message.

## What is Speech Sound Disorder (SSD)?

A small number of children have physical problems which mean that they are unable to make the sounds of speech. These include children with a cleft lip and/or palate. If your child has a cleft lip and/or palate, then they will be referred to a specialist team.

Most children have nothing physically different and yet still have problems saying and using sounds.

When children cannot say a sound on its own correctly after an adult, and are old enough to say that sound, they have an **Articulation Disorder.** This is usually a problem physically making the sound. For example, a child might say "sss" with the sound coming out of the side of the mouth, instead of the middle and so it doesn't sound correct to the listener.

Most problems with using clear speech are NOT caused by articulation disorder. Instead, the child has difficulties knowing how to use the sound in words. These mistakes happen even though the child can say the sound on its own. These are called **phonological disorders.**

Most people believe that Speech Sound Disorders are caused by physical problems with making sounds. This is true for articulation disorder, but **most speech sound problems are phonological.** This means that mouth exercises, correcting the child, or operations on their mouth, tongue, lips, or teeth would not help them. Many people have heard of being "tongue-tied." Unless this is so tight that it makes feeding difficult, this is **not** the cause of the child's speech sound problems. Instead, listening to words, thinking about how words are the same or different, and learning to use sounds in words to get the meaning across are much more likely to help. Children can have one of the following problems:

- **Phonological Delay.** The child makes mistakes that are seen in young children's speech.
- **Consistent Phonological Disorder.** The child makes mistakes that are unusual at any age.
- **Inconsistent Phonological Disorder.** The child says the same **word** differently each time they try to say it.

## Has bilingualism/multilingualism caused the Speech Sound Disorder?

No. There are no cases where bilingualism has caused a speech problem. In all cases the speech sound difficulty would have occurred no matter if the child had spoken one language or many languages. We know that lots of children have problems using clear speech and this is just as likely if the child speaks one language, two or more. **Deciding to use just one language will not help.** It is important to keep using your home language(s). These will help your child to understand their friends, siblings, relatives and wider community. Children who speak a home language are also better at learning the language of school, not worse!

The Speech and Language Therapist/Pathologist is likely to set home practice. You will practice sounds, words and games with your child in your home language(s).

## Will the speech sound errors be the same in both/all languages?

If your child has an articulation disorder, the mistake can be heard when the child says the sound on its own, and in words. This is likely to happen in both/all languages that they speak.

If your child has a phonological problem, then they will have no difficulties saying the sound on its own. However, in words, they will change the sound for another sound. You may think that the child is being lazy and cannot be bothered to use the sound in words. This is not true. Your child is not yet able to realise that they are using the wrong sound in words and spoken sentences.

You may notice different mistakes in the home language than in the mainstream language/ language of school. This is to be expected.

## What is the best treatment?

It is very important that you keep speaking your home language(s). These will have clear examples of words for your child to listen to. Learning your home language will help your child learn additional languages.

The Speech and Language Therapist/Pathologist will assess and provide treatment in home language. They will do this if they speak your language, or with the help of an interpreter if they do not speak your language.

Your child will also be referred for a hearing check.

Depending on the type of problem, your child may practice listening to and saying sounds, words and spoken sentences. This will be done through a series of lessons and games to make the work enjoyable. Children learn best when the games are fun.

It is important:

- not to correct your child's speech sound mistakes (unless the Speech and Language Therapist/Pathologist tell you to, using a helpful method such as a sound picture)
- not to tell them off and not to punish them if they make speech sound mistakes. Children do not realise they are making mistakes, even if it seems very obvious to an adult or other child.

- to make sure children and other adults do not correct your child, or be unkind to your child when they use unclear words or make mistakes with sounds.
- to help others in the family to understand Speech Sound Disorder by sharing this leaflet and video.
- to say words clearly in your home language so your child can hear lots of examples of how words are said.
- to encourage your child and to reward them with smiles, hugs and praise when they try hard or improve.
- to practice any games, activities or exercises as often as the Speech and Language Therapist/Pathologist recommends in home language(s). This is usually every day.

## Other problems

Some children will just have problems with sounds and saying words clearly. Other children may have difficulties with either understanding and using spoken language or both (Language Difficulty or Developmental Language Disorder). Some children don't recognise as many words as other children their age do (restricted vocabulary). Your child may need further assessments and treatments for other aspects of their speech, language, and communication.

## Ways you can help the speech and language therapist/pathologist

Do you notice words that your child regularly has problems saying clearly? Write these words down, or, if that is difficult, take a photo of the thing your child cannot say with your smartphone.

With permission, video any information your Speech and Language Therapist/Pathologist gives you by videoing the interpreter on your smartphone. Video any activities, games or exercises that the Speech and Language Therapist/Pathologist demonstrates so you can check that you are doing them correctly at home. That way you can listen/watch again and encourage people who know your child but couldn't be at the appointment to watch as well. That way, everyone will know what to do.

Even if you speak the same language as the Speech and Language Therapist/Pathologist, it is important to work with the interpreter. The interpreter will help your child work with the Speech and Language Therapist/Pathologist.

Finally, if you are not sure about anything that you have been told, ask questions. The Speech and Language Therapist and Interpreter are there to help you, your family, and your child.

*This leaflet was written by Dr Sean Pert, Consultant Speech and Language Therapist and Adviser on Bilingualism for the Royal College of Speech and Language Therapists, UK. The advice is based on evidence-based research, clinical experience, and professional guidelines.*

# Bilingual children with speech, language, and communication needs

*Notes for the Speech and Language Therapist/Pathologist:*

☑ Please ask an interpreter to provide the following information in the family's home language(s).

☑ Consider that some technical terms, including "sound," "word," "vocal tract," etc., may not have translation equivalents and will need examples to explain these clearly. Discuss these in the planning session before you discuss the diagnosis with the family.

☑ With permission from the interpreter, video and/or audio record the interpreter delivering this information in home language(s) and upload the recording so that it is available online (Generic information leaflets are not confidential information).

☑ Link the web address to a QR code and add it here with the language(s) available for quick access by the parent(s)/carer and family via a camera on a smartphone or tablet.

## Has using two or more language caused my child's speech, language, or communication needs?

No. There are no cases where a child or young person has experienced a speech, language, or communication need because they are bilingual or multilingual. Speaking two or more language is more common across the world than just speaking one language. Speaking two or more languages will not slow down the treatment, and will not make the speech, language, or communication need any worse.

## Should I stop speaking my home language(s) to help my child?

No. Speaking your home language(s) is very important and helps your child to learn how to communicate with their friends, siblings, relatives and others in their community. If they miss the chance to learn their home language in the early years, they will likely find it very difficult to learn later in life and may speak your home language in a way that is not as good as if they learn it now.

We know that many parent(s)/carers think that switching to just using the mainstream language (typically English) will help them to succeed at school. This is not true. Children who speak their home language are able to learn the language of education very easily.

We know that if parent(s)/carers switch to the mainstream language (typically English), then the child is very likely to lose their home language. This causes problems as they may not be able to speak to one or more of their parents, and the extended family.

Try to imagine your child at 18 years of age. Do you want him/her to be able to speak to you, the family, and members in the community, as well as being able to speak the mainstream language (typically English) confidently? If the answer is "yes," then you should speak your home language(s) to your child.

## Won't my child find learning two or more languages even harder because s/he has a speech, language, or communication need?

Young children find it much easier to learn to speak their home language(s) simply by hearing it and using it in everyday life. Even children with very severe speech, language, and communication needs can learn two or more languages. This is because children enjoy speaking to others and will naturally use the language that person speaks.

The more knowledge your child has of their home language(s), the easier it is for them to learn additional languages.

## Why should I speak my home language to my child?

You speak your home language(s) extremely well, and this is a wonderful model for your child to copy and learn from. Speaking your home language comes naturally, and helps your child to understand your traditions, beliefs and way of life. It provides your child with a sense of identity and belonging.

Speaking just the mainstream language/language of education (typically English) will likely mean that your child will lose the ability to speak their home language(s) completely.

## Will my child be confused by speaking two or more languages together?

Most bilingual speakers codeswitch. That is, use words from two languages (or more) in one spoken sentence. This is perfectly natural and nothing to be worried about. Your child will be able to tell who is speaking which language from a young age. There are no examples where a child has been confused by hearing or using two or more languages together.

## I have been told by a professional that using two or more languages is harmful

If a teacher, doctor, nurse or other professional has told you that using two or more languages with your child will cause problems, then **they are wrong**. Many professionals, especially those who speak only one language are not properly educated about bilingualism/ multilingualism. Speech and Language Therapists/Pathologists and Linguists who study language have thoroughly researched this area. We can be sure that bilingualism or multilingualism is normal, found throughout the world, and does not cause speech, language, and communication problems in children.

If a professional says this to you in the future, the Speech and Language Therapist/ Pathologist can help them to understand the most up-to-date research so they can give people the correct advice, that bilingualism is an advantage.

*This leaflet was written by Dr Sean Pert, Consultant Speech and Language Therapist and Adviser on Bilingualism for the Royal College of Speech and Language Therapists, UK. The advice is based on evidence-based research, clinical experience, and professional guidelines.*

# SPEECH AND LANGUAGE THERAPY ASSESSMENT REPORT

Date:

Clinic/Base/Hospital Address:

Telephone:

Email and web address:

## Speech and language therapy Assessment report: Bilingual/multilingual child or young person

| | |
|---|---|
| **Re:** | |
| **Date of Birth:** | |
| **Age** (Year; Completed months): | |
| **Home address:** | |
| **Nursery/School/Educational Setting:** | |

**Report written by:**

**SLT NAME**

Consultant/Advanced/Highly Specialist/Senior/Speech and Language Therapist/Speech and Language Pathologist

Copies to:

☐ Parent(s)/Guardian

☐ GP/Doctor

☐ School Special Educational Needs Co-ordinator

☐ Audiology

☐ Case notes

## Summary

*Language(s) of assessment*

X is a bilingual/multilingual/child/young person who comes from a home where:

- A language/languages other than English/mainstream language is/are spoken.
- A home language or languages are spoken alongside English/mainstream language.

X is a bilingual/multilingual child/young person who attends a care/school/education setting where the following language(s) are spoken:

**X was assessed with the assistance of a professional interpreter. Please note that a professional interpreter should be involved in all interactions with this family.**

X was assessed in the following languages:

| | |
|---|---|
| **Home language(s):** | |
| **Mainstream language/Language of education:** | |
| **Other:** | |

*Assessment scores*

As normative data including age equivalents, percentile ranks, standard scores, and other measures are *typically based on a monolingual population*, it is not accurate or ethical to quote such scores for a child or young person who is exposed to two or more languages. This would result in a false comparison and a result which would disadvantage the child or young person culturally and linguistically.

For these reasons, **scores are not included in this assessment report.** Instead, as recommended by Speech and Language Therapy and Pathology professional bodies internationally (RCSLT, UK; ASHA, USA; Speech Pathology, Australia), professional judgement based on descriptive, culturally appropriate adapted assessments will be cited.

**Scores based on monolingual home language speakers, or bilingual speakers *where available* have been applied and highlighted as appropriate to this child or young person.**

Any gatekeepers for services, additional needs, resources etc. should note the above. Demanding standard scores in the same way as for monolingual children or similar for access to resources is an example of institutional racism. Speech and Language Therapists and Pathologists are unable to comply with such requests, as it would be a breach of professional practice. Using *unmodified* standardised assessments based on monolingual children could result in disciplinary action against the therapist for breach of their professional code.

**The Speech and Language Therapist or Pathologist who has completed this assessment report is trained in the culturally and linguistically appropriate assessment of bilingual and multilingual children and young people.**

**In my professional opinion** X presents with the following diagnosis/diagnoses:

*Severity*

In my expert opinion, X has profound/severe/moderate difficult in this area/domain when compared to a bilingual or multilingual child of the same age.

In my expert opinion, X has low average/average/high average/moderately high/extremely high abilities in this area/domain when compared to a bilingual or multilingual child of the same age.

## Diagnosis/Diagnoses by speech and language domain

*Language*

Language Difficulties
Speech, Language, and Communication Needs (SLCN)
Language Disorder
Developmental Language Disorder (DLD)
Language Disorder associated with X (where X is an associated biomedical condition; the biomedical condition does not imply causation).
Restricted vocabulary (limited or poor word recognition and limited naming)
Word Finding Difficulties (that is, there is a *significant difference* between relatively good listening vocabulary and limited naming vocabulary; the child knows words but cannot always retrieve them with ease)

*Speech*

Note that Speech Sound Disorder (SSD) is a category and is NOT a diagnosis.

X presents with:

*Articulation: single sound (phone) production and imitation*

Articulation Disorder (not stimulable for phones s/he should have acquired by this age)
Motor speech difficulties

*Phonology: word level production and above*

Phonology (word level Speech Sound Disorder)
Phonological Delay

Consistent Phonological Disorder

Inconsistent Phonological Disorder (IPD)

*Motor speech*

Childhood Apraxia of Speech/Developmental Verbal Dyspraxia (CAS/DVD) as Inconsistent Phonological Disorder has been ruled out due to lack of response to the Core Vocabulary Programme.

*Disorders of fluency*

Stammering (also known as Stuttering)

Cluttering/social communication difficulties/voice disorder.

*No diagnosis is applicable*

X's speech, language, and communication skills are now within normal limits for a child of their age and therefore speech and language therapy is no longer required.

X has achieved all the therapy aims set for this episode of care, and speech and language therapy is not required at present.

## Recommendations

I recommend that:

1. **A professional interpreter is involved in all discussion with this family to ensure that informed consent for any decisions or actions is gained.**
2. **A bilingual/multilingual classroom assistant/teaching assistant is available for the child or young person who speaks X and Y, and trained by the Speech and Language Therapist or Pathologist in the home language programme.**
3. **Therapy aims should be achieved in the home language before being attempted in English/the mainstream language.**
4. Aims from the attached care plan are incorporated into X's individual Education Heath and Care Plan (EHCP).
5. **Double the time should be allocated** compared to a monolingual child speaking English or the mainstream language, in order to achieve the same outcomes (equitable input). Allocating the same time and duration as for a monolingual speaking child is an example of institutional racism.

6. The attached home language therapy programme is carried out by bilingual/multilingual school staff and parent(s)/carer for 15-20-30-45-60 minutes **on a daily basis.** Please note that unless the programme is implemented on this basis, it is unlikely to be effective and intervention by the speech and language therapy team alone will not resolve the child's identified needs.

7. X is provided with a differentiated curriculum and adult support (Bilingual/Multilingual Classroom Assistant/Teaching Assistant) to enable him/her to access the curriculum and develop his/her home language skills in the classroom situation.

8. The school Special Educational Needs Co-ordinator refer X to an Educational Psychologist for an assessment of his/her non-verbal learning skills with cultural and home language support and adaptation.

9. No recommendations are required at this time.

## Actions

*Onward referrals*

X has been referred to the Audiology service for a hearing assessment with parental permission.

X has been referred to the Regional Cleft Lip and Palate Team for an assessment with parental permission.

X has been referred to the Ear, Nose and Throat (ENT) for an assessment.

Therapy has been arranged with parental permission.

X has been referred to a Geneticist for an assessment with parental permission.

**Please note that the family will require a professional interpreter for the above appointment(s).**

*Actions*

A care plan and therapy programme has been set and are attached. Therapy aims will be reviewed at the end of this episode of care, or on request if X has achieved the therapy aims.

X's speech, language, and communication needs are expected to resolve, and so s/he has been discharged from the service. Please re-refer should there be any concerns in the future.

X's speech, language, and communication skills are within normal limits, and so s/he has been discharged from the service. Please re-refer should there be any concerns in the future.

## Background

For the current episode of care, this child was referred to me by (PERSON) on (DATE). S/he has been seen for X assessment appointments and X therapy sessions.

## Vocabulary – listening vocabulary

Listening vocabulary is the child's knowledge of words and ability to recognise words.

X was assessed using the Y. Date of assessment: dd/mm/yyyy; age on assessment: YY;MM.

## Vocabulary – naming vocabulary

X was assessed using the Y. Date of assessment: dd/mm/yyyy; age on assessment: YY;MM.

## Speech sounds (articulation and phonology)

X was assessed using the Y. Date of assessment: dd/mm/yyyy; age on assessment: YY;MM.

*Articulation*

Articulation is the ability to physically produce sounds in isolation. A child may have difficulties producing a sound for physical reasons, such as missing teeth, or because they have not learnt how to make the sound.

**ADD SOUND INVENTORY FOR THE HOME LANGUAGE HERE**

## English speech sounds

*Articulation: sound level*

X could produce the following sounds of English as **single sounds** even after a model provided by an adult speaker:

- Plosives (short sounds)
  p, b, t, d, k and g

- Fricatives (long sounds)

    f, v, s, z, "sh," and "zh" (as in "**sh**ell" and "trea**s**ure," respectively)
- Nasals (made with air coming out of the nose)

    m, n, and "ng" (as in "lu**ng**")
- Approximants

    w, l, "y" (as in "**y**ellow"), and "r" (as in "**r**abbit").

X had could *not* produce the following sounds of English as **single sounds** even after a model provided by an adult speaker:

- Plosives (short sounds)
    - p ➜ ""
    - b ➜ ""
    - t ➜ ""
    - d ➜ ""
    - k ➜ ""
    - g ➜ ""
- Fricatives (long sounds)
    - f ➜ ""
    - v ➜ ""
    - s ➜ ""
    - z ➜ ""
    - sh ➜ ""
    - zh (as in "trea**s**ure") ➜ ""
- Nasals (made with air coming out of the nose)
    - m ➜ ""
    - n ➜ ""
    - "ng" (as in "lu**ng**") ➜ ""
- Approximants
    - w ➜ ""
    - l ➜ ""
    - "y" (as in "**y**ellow") ➜ ""
    - "r" (as in "**r**abbit") ➜ ""

*Phonology: word level and above*

Phonology assessment examines "the ability to use sounds in context" (Dodd et al., 2002, p. 7). That is, using the sounds in real words. A child may be able to say a sound in isolation (articulate the sound) but not yet use it in words. This is termed phonological disorder.

**ADD PHONOLOGICAL INVENTORY FOR THE HOME LANGUAGE HERE**

X's speech contains error patterns. These error patterns reduce the contrast in X's speech sound system, making more words sound alike and therefore X's speech less intelligible.

*Delayed error patterns*

Y of X's speech error patterns are delayed. This means that the patterns are found in the speech of children younger than X.

**Note that for bilingual/multilingual children, age norms for English will not apply.**

The following delayed error patterns were identified in X's speech:

- Gliding – This is when the sounds "w," "l," "r," and "y" are confused.
- Deaffrication – This is when the affricates "ch"/"tch" (as in "chocolate" and "watch") and "dg"/"j" (as in "jigsaw" and "badge") are produced as just a short sound "t" and "d," respectively.
- Cluster reduction – This is when a word starting with two or three consonants is produced with fewer consonants, e.g., "**sp**oon," "**spr**ay," or "**br**ick."
  Please note that the second segment of s-clusters in English are unaspirated and perceived as *voiced* segments and so when cluster reduction is present it may *appear* that context sensitive voicing (CSV) is also present, but this is not the case. For example, "spider"/ˈsbaɪ.də/realised as [baɪdə] is cluster reduction *only*, **not** CSV.
- Fronting of velars – This is when sounds produced at the back of the mouth, that is, "k," "g," and "ng" (as in "lu**ng**") are realised as sounds made at the front of the mouth, typically, "t," "d," and "n," respectively.
- Weak syllable deletion – This is when a word with an unstressed syllable is produced without that syllable, e.g., "tomato" ➔ "mato."
- Stopping of fricatives – This is when a long sound such as "s" is produced as a short sound such as "t," so words such as "sock" are produced as "tock" or "dock."

- Context Sensitive Voicing - This is when a quiet sound such as "p" is produced as a loud sound such as "b" *before the vowel* (prevocalic), or a loud sound is produced as a quiet sound *after the vowel* (postvocalic).
- Final consonant deletion - Present in the speech of children aged less than two years, this is when the final sound is missed off a word. (This should not be confused with glottal stops, which are typical in several regional UK accents, including northern English accents).

UNUSUAL ERROR PATTERNS

Z of X's error patterns are unusual. This means that they do not occur in younger children's speech.

**Please note that some sounds patterns deemed unusual for English may be typical for children from a bilingual or multilingual background.**

The following unusual error patterns were identified in X's speech:

- Backing - when a sound made at the front is made at the back of the mouth. Typically, "t" and "d" are produced as "k" and "g," respectively.
- Affrication - when a sound is produced as an affrication (a long and short sound together).
- Initial consonant deletion - when the first sound of a word is missed off.
- Medial consonant deletion - when the middle sound of a word is missed off. (This should not be confused with glottal stops, which are typical in northern English accents).
- Intrusive consonant - when an additional sound is added.
- Denasalisation - when a sound is produced with air coming from the nose when it should be produced with air just coming out of the mouth
- Sound preference substitution - when the child uses a particular sound for a range of other sounds.

*Phonological awareness skills*

Phonological awareness is the ability to compare and contrast words and break words down into smaller chunks such as syllables, onset-rime, and single sounds.

X was assessed using the Preschool and Primary Inventory of Phonological Awareness. Date of assessment: dd/mm/yyyy; age on assessment: YY;MM.

Table X. Preschool and Primary Inventory of Phonological Awareness (PIPA)

| Sub-test | Comments: Scores not available for bilingual/multilingual children and young people | Comment |
|---|---|---|
| Syllable segmentation | | Extremely low/moderately low/low average/high average/moderately high/extremely high score |
| Rhyme awareness | | Extremely low/moderately low/low average/high average/moderately high/extremely high score |
| Alliteration awareness | | Extremely low/moderately low/low average/high average/moderately high/extremely high score |
| Phoneme isolation | | Extremely low/moderately low/low average/high average/moderately high/extremely high score |
| Phoneme segmentation | | Extremely low/moderately low/low average/high average/moderately high/extremely high score |
| Letter knowledge | | Extremely low/moderately low/low average/high average/moderately high/extremely high score |

## LIST INFORMAL AND ADAPTED ASSESSMENTS USED IN THE ASSESSMENT HERE

## Reference

Dodd, B., Hua, Zhu, Crosbie, S., Holm, A., & Ozanne, A. (2002). *Diagnostic evaluation of articulation and phonology*. Pearson. http://www.pearsonclinical.co.uk

## Professional organisations' bilingualism and multilingual pages

- **Royal College of Speech and Language Therapists (RCSLT)**
  Bilingualism: Guidance, resources and opportunities to support you in your role as a speech and language therapist working with bilingual clients.
  - www.rcslt.org/members/clinical-guidance/bilingualism/
    (Member log-in required for the unabridged version)
  - Bilingualism – Main learning points
    www.rcslt.org/wp-content/uploads/media/Project/RCSLT/1main-learning-points.pdf
  - SLT Assessment and Intervention: Best practice for children and young people in bilingual settings. Carol Stow and Sean Pert.
    www.rcslt.org/wp-content/uploads/media/Project/RCSLT/best-practice-cyp-bilingual-settings.pdf
- **American Speech-Language-Hearing Association (ASHA)**
  - Learning Two Languages www.asha.org/public/speech/development/learning-two-languages/
  - Bilingual Service Delivery
    www.asha.org/practice-portal/professional-issues/bilingual-service-delivery/
  - Dynamic Assessment by Dr Elizabeth Peña
    www.asha.org/practice/multicultural/dynamic-assessment/
- **Centre for Literacy and Multilingualism (CeLM), University of Reading**
  CeLM brings together a multidisciplinary group of researchers broadly interested in language, literacy and multilingualism.
  https://research.reading.ac.uk/celm/
- **National Association for Language Development in the Curriculum (NALDIC)**
  The national subject association for English as an Additional Language (EAL)
  https://naldic.org.uk

## Podcasts and videos

- **BBC Tiny Happy People**
  Bilingual babies: Your questions answered by a speech and language therapist

Speech and Language Therapist Monal Gajjar talks about bringing up bilingual children and answers some of parents' most common questions.

www.bbc.co.uk/tiny-happy-people/multiple-languages-slt/zj8fxbk

- **Kletsheads**

  The podcast about bilingual children for parents, teachers and speech and language therapists

  https://kletsheadspodcast.org

- **RCSLT Official**

  Developmental Language Disorder (DLD) – when is a diagnosis appropriate?

  DLD in a bilingual context, presented by Dr Sean Pert

  https://youtu.be/8uMOgNQCZrM

## Advice leaflets

- **Afasic**

  Bilingualism by Dr Sean Pert (2016)

  https://afasic.org.uk/download/28/

- **National Literacy Trust**

  Understanding multilingualism in the early years

  https://literacytrust.org.uk/resources/understanding-multilingualism-early-years/

  Including a range of leaflets and Bilingual quick tips in 19 languages:

  https://literacytrust.org.uk/early-years/bilingual-quick-tips/

- **Guy's & St Thomas' Children & Young People's Community Speech & Language Therapy Service**

  Keep your language alive: A helpful guide to early language development

  www.evelinalondon.nhs.uk/resources/patient-information/community-slt-language-guide-bilingual.pdf

## Books on bilingualism

- Multilingual Matters

  www.multilingual-matters.com

- Baker, C. (2000). *A parents' and teachers' guide to bilingualism*. Multilingual Matters Ltd. ISBN: 9781783091607

- Cunningham, U. (2020). *Growing up with two languages: A practical guide for multilingual families and those who support them*. Routledge. ISBN 9780815380566

## SLT web sites

- Bilingualism is an advantage
  www.bilingualism.co.uk
- Bilingualism London Clinical Excellence Network
  www.bilingualismcen.com

## Bilingual assessments and interventions

- **Functional Language Across Countries (FLAC)**
  Polish, Spanish, Slovak, Lithuanian, Russian, and Mandarin. Published by Black Sheet Press
  www.blacksheeppress.co.uk/product-category/speech-and-language-therapy/multilingual-resources/bilingual-assessments-multilingual-resources/

- **Bilingual Speech Sound Screen (BiSSS)**
  Revised and expanded edition: Pakistani heritage languages, Mirpuri, Punjabi and Urdu. Download version. By Dr Carol Stow and Dr Sean Pert. Published by the University of Manchester.
  https://estore.manchester.ac.uk/product-catalogue/faculty-of-biology-medicine-and-health/school-of-health-sciences/bilingual-speech-sound-screen-bisss/bilingual-speech-sound-screen-bisss

- **Bilingual Assessment of Simple Sentences (BASS)**
  An expressive language screening assessment of early sentence production for children with a Pakistani-heritage background speaking Mirpuri, Punjabi, or Urdu as a home language in the UK. By Dr Sean Pert and Dr Carol Stow. Published by the Royal College of Speech and Language Therapists.
  www.rcslt.org/members/clinical-guidance/bilingualism/bilingualism-learning/bilingualism-bass/ (Member log-in required or contact via www.rcslt.org/help-and-support/contact-us/)

- **Adaptations of the MacArthur-Bates Communicative Development Inventories (MB-CDIs)**
  Parent report instruments which capture important information about children's developing abilities in early language, including vocabulary, comprehension, production, gestures, and grammar.
  Adaptations of the MacArthur-Bates CDIs have been developed in a number of languages other than American English, including separate versions for dialects which are

sufficiently different to merit alternate instruments. The authors of each adaptation version should be contacted directly for information.

https://mb-cdi.stanford.edu/adaptations.html

- **Language Intervention in the Early Years (LIVELY)**
  A research project funded by the Heather van der Lely Foundation which aims to compare the effectiveness of language interventions for children with Language Difficulties (McKean, C., Jack, C., Ashton, E., Preston, E., Benson, K., Rose, N., Letts, C., Stringer, H., Wareham, H., Pert, S. & Trebacz, A.).
  Adaptations of the *Building Early Sentences Therapy* (BEST) (McKean et al., 2013) in Polish, Sylheti, and Mirpuri are in press.
  https://research.ncl.ac.uk/lively/

## Computer tools for analysing expressive language automatically, such as Mean Length of Utterance (MLU)

- Computerized Language ANalysis (CLAN) by Leonid Spektor, Carnegie Mellon University
  https://dali.talkbank.org/clan/
  - Manual by Brian MacWhinney (2022)
  https://talkbank.org/manuals/CLAN.pdf
- See this open access paper on using computer analysis in speech and language therapy assessment
  Pezold, M. J., Imgrund, C. M., & Storkel, H. L. (2020). Using computer programs for language sample analysis. *Language, Speech & Hearing Services in Schools, 51*, 103–114.
  https://doi.org/10.1044/2019_LSHSS-18-0148

## Information on languages

- **Ethnologue: Languages of the World**
  www.ethnologue.com

## The IPA chart and ear-training

- **Seeing Speech**
  Lawson, E., Stuart-Smith, J., Scobbie, J. M., & Nakai, S. (2018). *Seeing speech: an articulatory web resource for the study of phonetics*. University of Glasgow. Retrieved April 22, 2022, from www.seeingspeech.ac.uk/

# Index